DITCHING  DRIVE-THRU

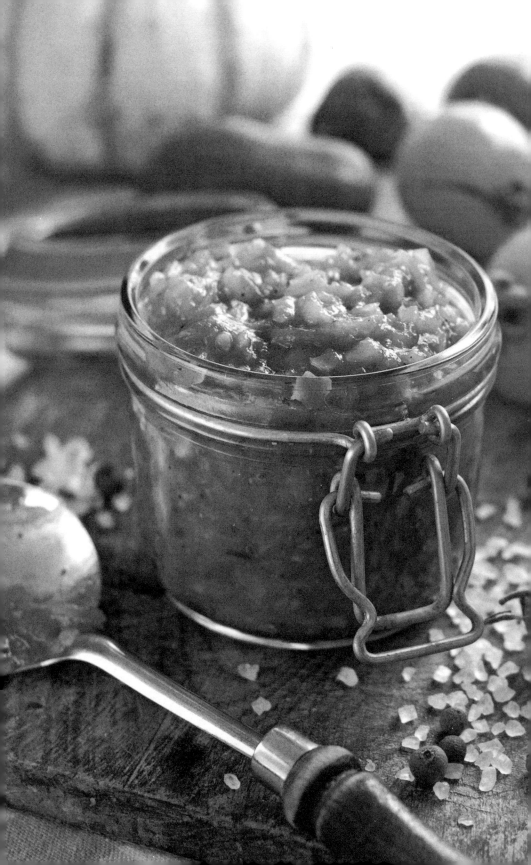

DITCHING (THE) DRIVE-THRU

HOW TO
PASS UP PROCESSED FOODS,
BUY FARM FRESH,
AND TRANSFORM YOUR FAMILY'S EATING HABITS
ON A MODERN MOM'S SCHEDULE

J. NATALIE WINCH

SPIKEHORN PRESS
AUSTIN, TEXAS

DITCHING THE DRIVE-THRU

Copyright © 2015, J. Natalie Winch

Spikehorn Press
4029 Guadalupe St.
Austin, Texas 78751 U.S.A.
512-220-0544
mailbox@spikehornpress.com • *www.spikehornpress.com*

Printed in the United States of America

Front cover photography © Okea/iStock/Thinkstock
Interior photograph credits © Thinkstock *ii, vi, viii*, 2, 12, 21, 28, 38, 54, 70, 79, 84, 92, 96, 107, 110, 117, 124, 154, 156-160

Publisher's Cataloging-in-Publication
Winch, J. Natalie.
    Ditching the drive-thru : how to pass up processed foods, buy farm fresh, and
        transform you family's eating habits on a modern mom's schedule /
        J. Natalie Winch ; foreword by Joel Salatin.
        pages cm
    Includes bibliographical references and index.
    LCCN 2015940352
    ISBN 978-1-943015-06-1
    ISBN 978-1-943015-07-8 (ebook)
    1. Natural foods. 2. Food habits. 3. Nutrition. I. Title.

TX369.W56   2015   641.3'02
                         QBI15-600102

DEDICATION

In memory of my grandmothers:
Esther Cantor Gaffin
and
Emily Gillman Savage

and

In honor of small family farms
and sustainable food producers.

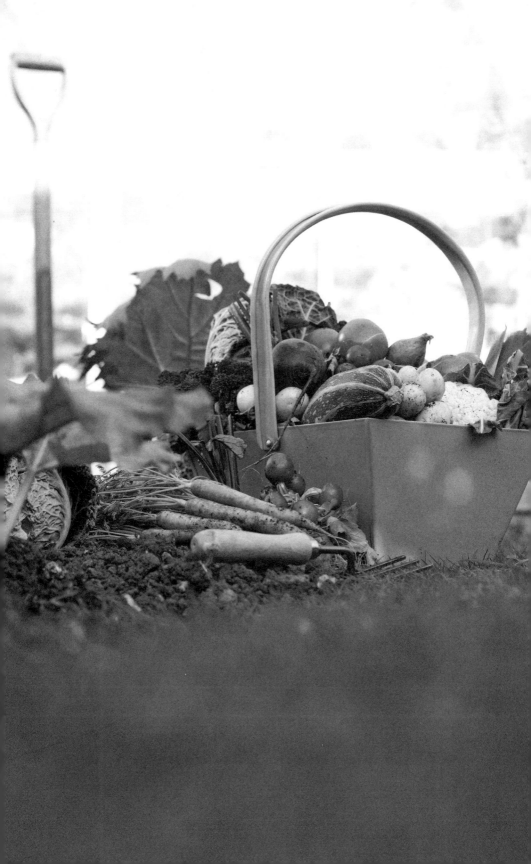

TABLE OF CONTENTS

Acknowledgments   IX

Foreword   XI

Preface   XV

PART I THE CALL FOR CHANGE:
MODERN AMERICA'S RELATIONSHIP WITH FOOD

1 Food, Culture, and Perception: Sisyphus Vs. Zeus   3

2 Diet Mythology: Faith in Food   13

3 The Food Maze: Seeing the Boundaries   29

4 Corporate Marketing Manipulation: Context Creates Story   39

5 Reading the Compass: Making Informed Choices   55

PART II EMBARKING ON THE JOURNEY:
HOW TO MAKE A CHANGE THAT LASTS

6 The Value of Farm-Fresh: Looking Beyond the Wallet   71

7 Agri-cabulary: The Language of Dealing Direct   85

8 Navigation: Keeping Sane on the Journey   97

9 Perpetuation: Creating and Maintaining Good Habits   111

10 Taking the First Step: Turning Theory into Practice   125

Epilogue   137

Appendix A: The Thirty-Month Plan
     and Why You Need One   141

Appendix B: Food Preservation and Recipes   151

Resources   162

Selected Bibliography   165

Index   169

About the Author   173

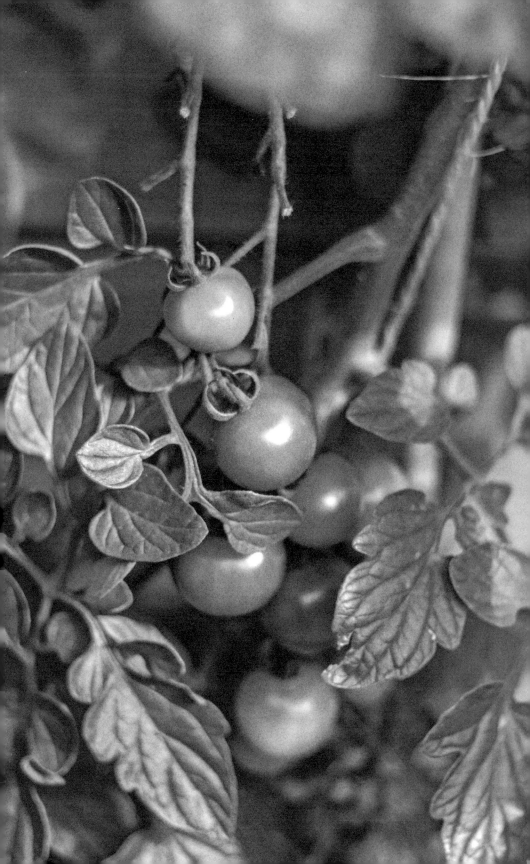

Acknowledgments

Many people inspired me to jot down the information provided in these pages in the hopes that it could help others move forward in their attempts to escape the industrial food merry-go-round. Without the constant encouragement of my husband, Greg, none of this would have come to fruition. When I broke my ankle a few years ago, he suggested that I finally take the time to work on that book I'd always talked about writing. Divine Providence always has a plan, and maybe I needed to break my ankle so that I would be forced to actually sit down and think things through for a couple of weeks. Without Greg's encouragement, I would have just sat around, watched bad TV, and been miserable.

I would also like to thank my children, Maddy and Seamus, who patiently realized that there were hours I needed in order to get this project completed. My children are the center of my universe and they know it, but they were able to let something else become my focus for a short time, which I genuinely appreciate.

My friend and coworker Sherrie Erikson was critical in the process and ideology of this project. She spent hours considering the work and inspired the Thirty-Month Plan.

Whether they realize it or not, Joel Salatin and Mark and Mary-ann Nolt were pivotal in the completion of this manuscript. Every trip to the Nolts' farm is a learning experience for me. From the first trip, when Maryann explained their transition from conventional farming to grass-based farming, to our last trip, when we discussed sourdough starters, I have always come away with new insights and inspirations. Their farm is also where I purchased Joel Salatin's book *Everything I Want to Do is Illegal*, which explains the farmer's predicament in the current food system. I wrote to Mr. Salatin for permission to use excerpts from his book to teach my English classes. His positive response to my letter, and subsequent publishing of excerpts from that letter, gave me the literary confidence to take the information I was disseminating in my classroom, expand it, and put it out to the public.

My parents, my in-laws, and their parents before them instilled in me the importance of tradition. I would be remiss if I did not acknowledge the enormous impact this had on my worldview and who I am today. From them I learned that I shouldn't "throw the baby out with the bath water," that while new methods and ideas may seem better, they do not negate the old way of doing things, and that we should evaluate ideas with an open mind before just jumping on a bandwagon.

I would also like to thank Mary Jane Chambers (my co-teacher), Laura Oakes (my former supervisor), and the students of my Contemporary Studies classes of 2010, 2011, and 2012, my first three years of teaching a curricular unit called "The Politics of Food." Without their interest, enthusiasm, and probing questions, I may not have seen the need for a manuscript of this type—one that keeps the information accessible and on point!

Lastly, I would like to thank Fred Walters for giving me a chance, and the entire team at Acres U.S.A. for helping me make this book a reality. I can't thank Amanda Irle enough for her help, guidance, and patience throughout the process of putting this book together. Her expertise not only helped me become a better writer, but a better teacher of writing.

Foreword

Joel Salatin is a third-generation farmer whose family owns and operates Polyface Farm in Virginia's Shenandoah Valley. He is the author of many books, including Everything I Want to Do Is Illegal *and* Folks, This Ain't Normal, *and has been featured in Michael Pollan's* New York Times *bestseller* The Omnivore's Dilemma *and the award-winning documentary* Food, Inc.

Every time I talk to a group about getting in touch with their food supply, healing the planet one bite at a time, or cultivating enthusiasm for domestic culinary arts—all common sound bites—I receive thunderous applause and then . . . then the queries and excuses start:

"I don't have the time."

"I don't have the money."

"I don't know how to cook."

"I don't have a freezer."

"I don't have a canner."

"How do I know if a farmer is honest?"

"How do I know unpackaged food is safe?"

"My kids are picky eaters."

The script plays out every time, on every socioeconomic level, in every geographic region. Our modern American culture, with its addiction to supermarkets, take-out, pop-n-serve, and government food pontification, is profoundly ignorant about eating. You'd think something as commonplace as eating would yield sophisticated understanding, yea, even professional-level knowledge among the populace.

But alas and alack, most modern Americans demean and cheapen body fuel to a mundane afterthought, less than a comma in our helter-skelter, plugged-in, harried lives. Running on dirty fuel, our people now lead the world in per capita health care costs, all the while spending the least—in both money and time—on food. Leading the world in health costs and cheap food may not be a good thing.

Our fixation on food is palpable, confirmed by the proliferation of cooking shows and the Food Channel's success. But too much of this is a spectator sport. More of us need to get into the game and participate. Intimidated by cooking's seeming complexity and the whole-food enigma—after all, a can of processed Harvard beets looks quite different than a fresh beet acquired from the patio pot garden, with roots and top and full orb fletched with soil—too many people yearning to do better settle for vicarious reading and watching.

It's time to leave the sidelines. It's time to play the game. Natalie Winch is both mentor and coach. A more perfect example of middle-class America could not exist. Yet this New Jersey high school English teacher, with husband and two children—what could be more typical?—creates a plan as simple and fundamental as a shopping list. Applying the most tried-and-true goal-setting templates to the traditional heart of the home, Winch takes us on a delightful journey—along with her beloved Homer's *Odyssey* as metaphor—and leaves us empowered to exit our bleacher seat, charging onto the field, game plan in hand.

As a farmer raising nutrient-dense, land-healing pastured livestock and poultry for thousands of urban householders, I yearn for Natalie's can-do empowerment to be more widely adopted. For farmers like me, desperate for enough customers to make their farms economically and emotionally viable, I want to hold Natalie up on a pedestal as an icon of successful domestic eating. Here she is, maven of familial food integrity.

What makes her saga even more special is that she's not a scientist, food nutritionist, or gourmand. She didn't wait for a grant or a reality TV show offer. She started where most of these stories start—how can I be a better mom for my kid? It's really that simple. This is not about guilt as much as it is about liberating ourselves from the bondage of shallow, nutrient-deficient, pseudo-food-like fuel for our bodies.

The current food and farming situation in our country is a physical manifestation of the cumulative choices made prior to today. In twenty years, the same will be true. I can guarantee that if thousands adopted Natalie's philosophy and practice, the world our grandchildren inherit will be decidedly different—and better—than the one we live in today.

Who else but a high school English teacher, searching for a metaphor to describe a despicable industrial-mechanical food system, would choose the cyclops? I laughed out loud, realizing that Natalie, who doesn't have a house full of gourmet foodie magazines, brings a fresh perspective to the better dining conundrum. Under her practical tutelage, excuses fall away . . . one by one.

So if you want to walk instead of talk. If you want to do instead of dream. If you want to play instead of observe. If you want to change instead of wish, here is a great little story to get you going on your own food empowerment odyssey. Here's to your legacy adventure.

JOEL SALATIN
JANUARY 2013

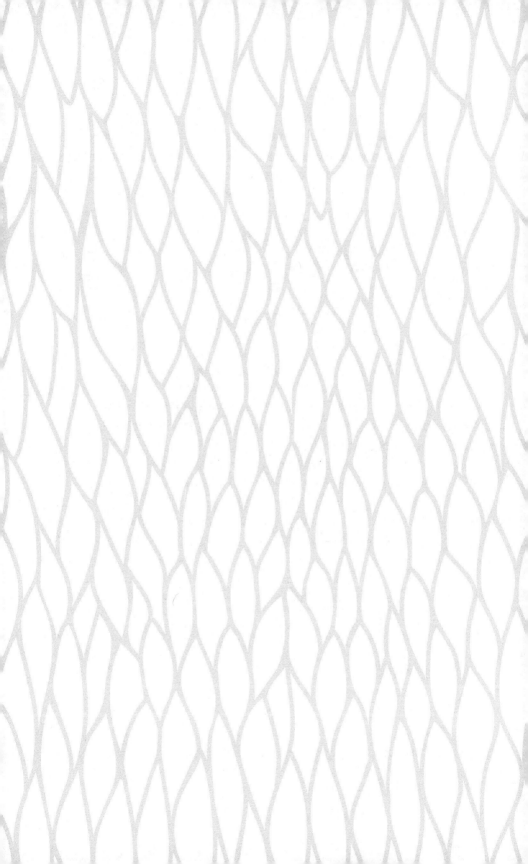

Preface

I am not a professional. But please attempt this at home!

This book is the story of my family's odyssey, our journey of learning about the food we eat and the course it takes from the farm to our plates. It is the compilation of a decade of research and experience, getting stuck in ruts, taking wrong turns, learning from our mistakes (well, some of them anyway), and trying to live life to the best of our abilities.

We are a healthy family of four living in a small town in southern New Jersey. I am an English teacher at a public high school. My husband, Greg, takes public transportation to his job as a professor at a state university in Philadelphia. My children attend the local public school. We are involved at our synagogue and enjoy spending time together as much as we are able (Greg and I are enjoying as much of this as possible—we know that the children's desire to spend most of their time with us will soon be over). While we are exposed to more germs than the average person (four schools' worth, plus the Philadelphia subway), we have fewer colds and haven't had the flu in years. And we aren't the types to constantly use hand sanitizer.

Even friends I have had for years will start apologizing for their grammar as soon as they remember what subject I teach. Similarly, people start making excuses or become defensive about their eating habits when I start "talking food." I talk about food because I love to eat. But this begs the question, why are so many people ashamed of how they eat? A colleague once asked me about community supported agriculture (CSA). When I explained how it worked—driving to the farm weekly to pick up my produce—she responded, "Well, that's fine for you, but what about the rest of us?" It's funny how perception works, because in my eyes, I am "the rest of us." How is driving to the farm once a week to pick up my produce any different from driving to the grocery store once a week? Actually it's very different—the people are generally very friendly, the produce is super fresh and pesticide-free, and there are no long checkout lines. Although I have to admit, I sometimes I miss reading the headlines from the *World News Weekly*.

I find food production inherently fascinating—we all eat, but most people don't seem to know where the food comes from. We don't like to associate steak with steer, or think about milk as the bodily fluid of a cow. Why are we afraid of the truth, the reality, of what our food really is, and where it begins its journey to our plates? The more I have learned about this, and just about everything else in life, as well, the more I realize how much more there is to learn. It's cliché, I know, but it is true. I have had the blessing of amazing teachers along this journey through life, who all had one ideology in common: knowledge is empowerment.

Before taking the first step of a long journey, it's important to know where you're starting out. You can't decide how to get to where you want to be unless you know where you are now! That's why this book is divided into two parts: the first tackles the current state of food in our culture and how it ties into the rise of now-ubiquitous health problems like obesity and diabetes. I also discuss some of the more troubling, lesser-known aspects of industrial farming, like concentrated animal feeding operations and pesticides. Part two reveals how you can fight the seeming omnipresence of the industrial food system and arms you with the practical knowledge you need to make informed decisions about what you feed yourself and your family. I'll give you tips on how to find a local farmer near you that will suit your needs, as well as explaining common terms and what to expect when shopping from small farms. I've also included strategies on planning meals and stocking your pantry so you can declare and maintain your independence from overprocessed, underflavored ready-to-eat or fast food meals. A roadmap of sorts is provided to you in Appendix A. The Thirty-Month Plan is intended to keep you from losing your way as you map out your own personal route to better eating and empowered choices.

When I joined my synagogue, my mother told me to get involved because "you will only get out of this experience what you are willing to put into it." That holds true for so many things in life. If for you food is only a matter of convenience, consuming enough calories to keep you going, no matter the physical consequences or quality of the calories you consume, then return this book. It is of no use to you. However, if you are willing, there is a world of wonder and good health just waiting for you. But nutritionally dense food is no longer convenient. You will have to work for it. And what we have learned is that most of the work is rethinking how we perceive our food. Do you want to let others control you, or do you want to take control? Are you willing to do the work? Remember, you will only get out of this what you put into it.

I'm not a nutritionist. I do not play one on TV. I have no formal training in medicine. I am a food enthusiast who has extensively researched my subject. I am a mother who is concerned about the health and well-being of my children. I am a member of the fast-paced American culture who feels overwhelmed by cultural expectations for myself and my children, overwhelmed by the volume and diversity of food choices and the sheer volume of information about that food. This book is a chronicle of how my family came to be where we are and what we learned along the way as well as a map to guide you on your own journey. I'll even tell you the moral of the story upfront (the proverbial string tied to the gate of the labyrinth): You have more control over the food you eat than you think.

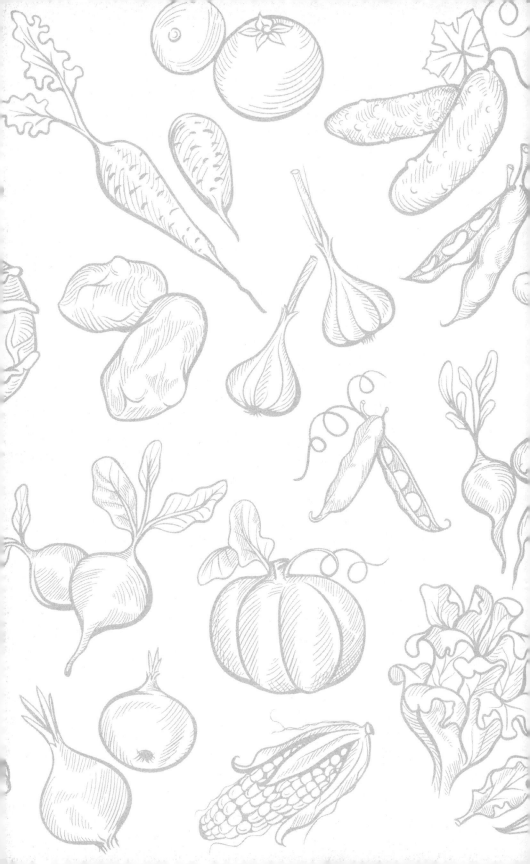

Part I

The Call for Change

MODERN AMERICA'S RELATIONSHIP WITH FOOD

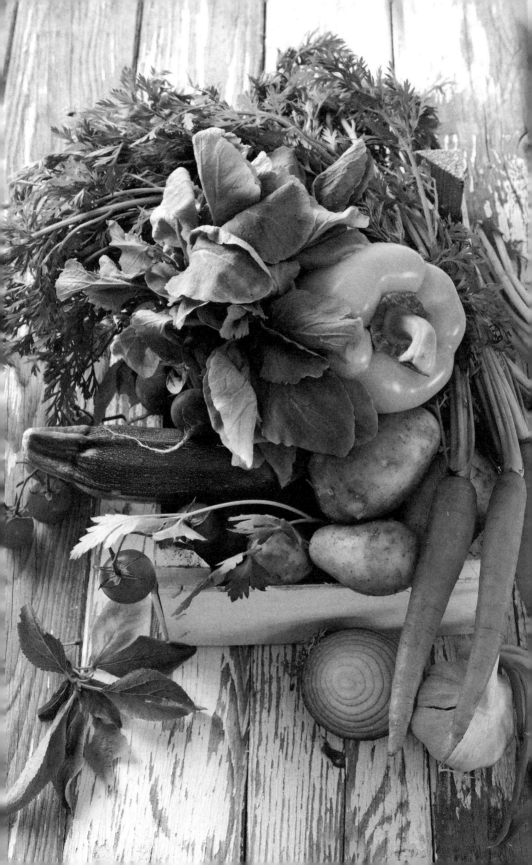

Food, Culture, and Perception

SISYPHUS VS. ZEUS

1

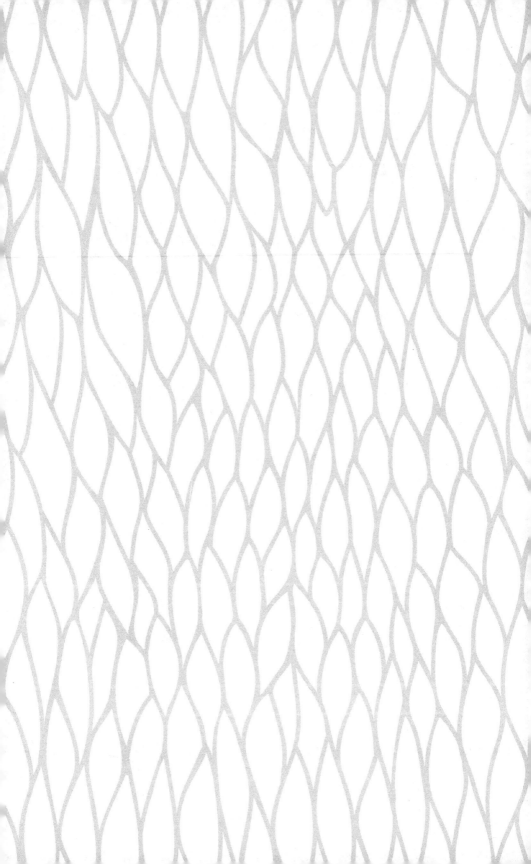

L ike many people, food has always been an important part of my life.

I'm Jewish. My parents raised my siblings and me in a kosher home. The laws of keeping kosher (kashrut) and the reasoning behind that the practice are beyond the scope of this book, but suffice it to say that dairy products and meat are not eaten at the same meal (and shouldn't touch the same plates, cookware, or utensils), and animals must be slaughtered in a humane and ritually specific way. When I was a child, I never considered any of this. All I knew was that I didn't eat cheeseburgers or bacon and, of course, I didn't eat bacon cheeseburgers! I knew that I was different from my friends because I couldn't eat what they ate—call it my first awareness of food.

I was blessed with a mother who was and still is an excellent cook, whose mother (may she rest in peace) was an amazing cook. Despite working outside the home Monday through Friday, my mom made us dinner every night, and almost every night the five of us sat down to dinner together. No TV. No phone calls. Just family and food from 6:15 to 7:00 every evening. We were busy, like any typical family. My brother and I played sports, my sister was a cheerleader, and we had Hebrew school for six hours a week. But we made it to the table, all five of us, most nights of the week. Don't think it was this idyllic *Leave It to Beaver* scene. We kicked each other under the table, made faces, showed chewed food, and pushed our luck until my dad was ready to blow his top. He would sit and drum his fingers on the table faster and faster until he eventually erupted. It usually took about three months; he never rushed into anything. But my family, the core of humanity that was most important to me, all sat together and ate a meal. This was pretty typical of the sixties and early seventies, at least where I grew up, because if I went to someone else's house for dinner, I experienced much the same thing.

Our regular family dinners had one of the largest impacts on me and my attitude toward food, not just the social benefits of the family meal, but having food that was cooked at home, by my very busy mother. Yes, she used frozen vegetables and we drank Tang and ate Quisp cereal for breakfast, and okay, the Tang probably had an ingredient list full of things I can't pronounce, but it was the sixties! If it was good enough for the astronauts, it was good enough for us. But Tang was the anomaly, since most of what we ate was made from scratch. I was unaware at the time of how this shaped my attitude about food, but looking back now, I realize that my mother is probably the reason sitting down to eat with my family has become such a priority in my home. And we do, as many nights a week as we can—no TV, no phones, no distractions from the outside world for about a half-hour.

I understand that many people do not see how they can accommodate homemade, nutritious, sit-down dinners every night, or even most nights. We live in a culture of busy. It's certainly not a misperception that you are busy. You are. The question is, in this time of increasingly innovative and amazing conveniences, why do we remain busier than any generation before us?

Nowadays, the most prevalent first-world occupations leave us with few to no tangible results of our labor. If you are an accountant, data-entry clerk, or a software engineer, you have nothing to hold in your hand at the end of an eight-hour workday. While these sorts of jobs can be emotionally fulfilling, if you're lucky, they just do not bear the same sense of accomplishment. We crave to see the fruits of our labors in tangible form; otherwise, however hard we work, we're left feeling like Sisyphus, forever pushing a boulder uphill but never getting anywhere.

I teach senior English. My students walk out of my classroom, never to be seen by me again (for the most part). While that is exactly how it should be, there is no closure or resolution in my job. Part of the thrill of home-canning for me is seeing the results of my day's work. I look over at the counter and see a row of jars lined up, cooling off. It is the polar opposite of my job, the results of which are completely intangible. Although my family does not entirely depend upon my canning abilities to get us through the winter, that fact does not diminish the sense of purpose that tangible line of jars instills. I can't help but think that we create busy-ness for ourselves in an attempt to compensate for the lack of unambiguous, discernible fruits of our labors.

Our consumerist culture is a beneficiary of our "too-busy-to-blank" perception of ourselves, so it's in the food industry's best interest to perpetuate the cycle. This attitude is the impetus for the exponential growth of the prepared and processed food market and plays to the quintessential American persona—go-getters out there going and getting. And the more we go, the more we get—and the more we end up paying for it in the end. The shift in American agriculture from small family farms to large corporate conglomerations has paralleled the growth of the processed, prepared-meal industry that works to produce cheap and easy food. As these changes occurred in agriculture and food production, our waistlines increased, as did the prevalence of things like heart disease and type 2 diabetes. Couple this growth with the average American's hectic schedule and a corporate desire to succeed and we find ourselves in our current cultural food turmoil: caught somewhere between farm-fresh healthy foods that doctors are recommending and the more readily accessible convenience foods.

I think one major problem with diet in America these days is our cultural propensity to associate pleasure with guilt. Some Zeus of the food industry decides that fat is bad for us and suddenly avoiding fat becomes a moral issue and our ability to do so a sign of our strength against temptation. People eat salads with no dressing, have a skinless, boneless (and usually tasteless) factory-raised chicken breast for dinner, and top it off with some fat-free ice cream. Like I said, I bought into it for a while, and I felt terribly guilty every time I got away from it. One of my favorite snacks is stovetop-popped popcorn, especially with either butter and cheese or butter and Tabasco sauce (don't make that face until you try it), and on an otherwise relaxing Sunday afternoon, watching a football game, grading some papers, and eating popcorn, I would feel bad about my butter indulgence. I would think about the foods I would skip in the coming day or week, or the extra workout or longer run I would endure in order to atone for my Sunday snack.

~~~~~~~~

The diet industry presents us with a simple equation: fat = unhealthy. Of course, it tends to ignore the possibility that increased body fat is related to the chemicals and additives in processed foods manufactured by the industrialized food system. Fat in itself is not inherently unhealthy, although fat-laden refined food generally is. As our food becomes more and more processed in order to make food easier and faster to consume, our people are growing less and less healthy. Food quality declines, overall health declines, people start gaining weight, and then the diet industry gets a major boost.

Discussing this recently, a friend told me that the actual number of Americans who are overweight has dropped over the past five years. I didn't believe her, so I looked it up. She was right: the number of Americans who are categorized as overweight has dropped. But that is a misleading statistic. While the number of people categorized as overweight did drop from 35.9 percent to 35.3 percent, the number of people classified as obese went up from 26.1 percent to 27.1 percent.[1] On CDC color-coded maps, one can see the maps go from mostly light yellow in 1994, meaning less than 14 percent of the population is obese, to the current maps where almost all states are red or dark red, meaning greater than 26 percent of the population is obese.[2] Fewer people fall into the overweight category because more and more people are edging their way into the obese category. Even more distressing, the number children who are obese or mortally obese is larger than the number of adults. This was so alarming to First Lady Michelle Obama that she made fighting childhood obesity her cause.

The number of children classified as obese or overweight has doubled in the past thirty years to 25 percent of the population under nineteen years of age.[3] Rather than investigating why this has happened over the last few years, we put our children on weight-loss diets as well. Why haven't more people made a connection between the increase in the number of processed foods available and the increase in childhood obesity?

My father recently gave me a textbook that belonged to my grandmother from her domestic science course in the Philadelphia public schools. We estimate that she took the course in about 1915 or so. In addition to instructions for maintaining a coal stove, sweeping a room, and doing laundry with a washboard, the book contains numerous chapters on food preparation before the days of refrigeration. The recommended diet was a balance of meat, dairy, and vegetables, with limited sweets. The book included instructions for making all meals from scratch, because there were no other options. And that was what my grandmother did, even though she worked full time outside the home.

In 1920, the same era as this textbook, 83 in 100,000 people died from cancer. In 2005, 189 people in 100,000 died from cancer. Other causes of death, like cardiovascular disease and pneumonia, have dropped in the same time period.[4] So why have deaths from cancer increased, even after all of the recent medical breakthroughs? In May of 2010, the President's Cancer Panel reported to President Barack Obama that "the true burden of environmentally induced cancers has been grossly underestimated."[5]

There were also changes in food production during the same time period. For example, after the Great Depression and Dust

Bowl era, we saw the rise of industrialized agriculture as families lost their farms. Later, in the boom of the 1950s, Americans had more and more convenience foods available, upon which we became increasingly dependent. Smaller family farms that once produced nutrient-dense foods were not as profitable for corporate moguls as large industrial farms that could supply the large quantities of raw materials to process into convenience foods. Last year, in one of my classes, a student insisted that the most valuable kitchen appliance is the microwave, a device that did not even exist at the time my grandmother's textbook was written. A microwave can be handy for reheating leftovers or frozen dinners, but you can't cook an entire meal from scratch with it. Could there be a link between these changes in the food we consume and these cancer rates? I don't know for certain, but maybe we need to learn to make time to prepare some of our own meals and see if that slows down this trend.

If you make an honest assessment of what makes food sense to you, which would you rather be eating? Food the way nature intended, with all of its available nutrients? Or food bought in a package with a mile-long list of unpronounceable ingredients? I understand the appeal of convenience, but most people with whom I engage in discussion on this subject tell me they don't know how to prepare nutritious homemade meals and keep up with their day-to-day lives. I'll give you some encouragement: it isn't that difficult. All you need is a little self-confidence and enough chutzpah to take a little baby-step out of your comfort zone.

NOTES

[1] Lindsay Sharp, "U.S. Obesity Rate Climbing in 2013," *Gallup*, November 1, 2013, http://www.gallup.com/poll/165671/obesity-rate-climbing-2013.aspx.

[2] "Maps of Trends in Diagnosed Diabetes and Obesity," Centers for Disease Control and Prevention, 2011, http://www.cdc.gov/diabetes/statistics.

[3] Immuno Laboratories, Inc., "Overweight and Obesity in Children," *Better Health USA*, July 10, 2010, http://www.betterhealthusa.com/public/227.cfm.

4 *Vital Statistics of the United States,* 1900–1970, U.S. Public Health Service, annual, Vol. I and Vol II; 1971–2001, U.S. National Center for Health Statistics, *Vital Statistics of the United States,* annual; *National Vital Statistics Report (NVSR)* (formerly *Monthly Vital Statistics Report)*; and unpublished data.

5 "Cancer and Toxic Chemicals," Physicians for Social Responsibility, http://www .psr.org/environment-and-health/confronting-toxics/cancer-and-toxic-chemicals. html (accessed August 24, 2014).

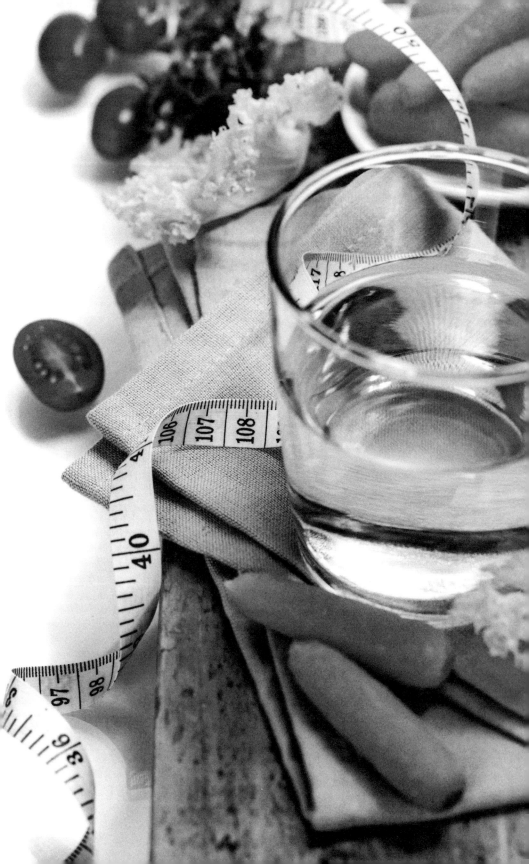

DIET MYTHOLOGY

FAITH IN FOOD

2

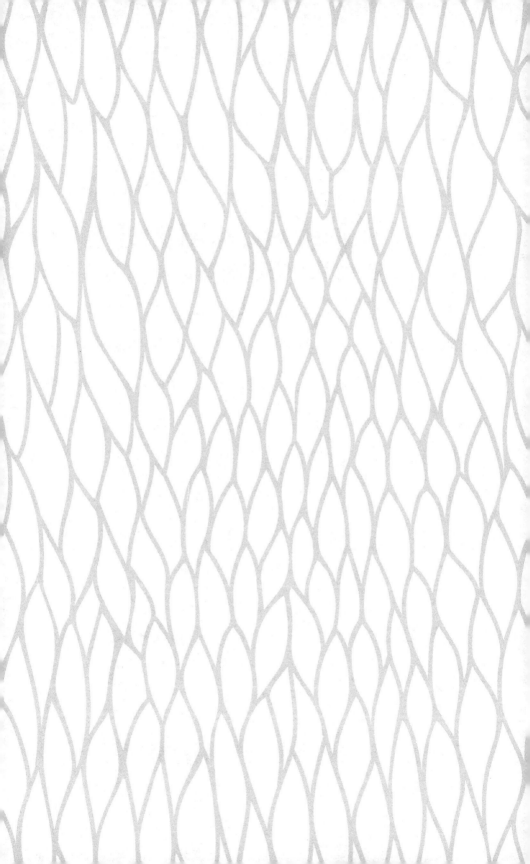

Diet and body image are inextricably linked, just like the economic structure surrounding our food and dietary supplements. Our culture feeds us an image of an unattainable body and face. Most of the bodies we see on TV or in advertisements have been, at the least, computer retouched, if not entirely computer-generated. I've retouched photos on my computer—it's really easy to erase that horrible zit or smooth away that frown line that cuts down the center of the forehead. I see exercise equipment touted by models with lean muscular bodies, bodies that may not even be real, and yet, because they are presented as real, and as some kind of ideal, many Americans see those advertisements and wonder if they would be happier if they had flatter abs or a firmer tushy. And then those words will echo in their minds, "Maybe I should go on a diet. . . ." Even people who are generally happy with their lives express their disgust about how they look. We don't have to worry about other people judging us—we do a great job of judging ourselves.

We are inundated by images of muscular people touting exercise equipment, and the fashion industry makes clothes for flag-poles, not people. The perceptions derived from advertising are a catalyst for distress about our bodies, a distress perpetuated by the medical community through this constant barrage of warnings about being overweight. The current ideal weight for a fifty-five-year-old woman who is five foot five is 126 pounds.[1] In 1911, when the obesity rate was less than 1 percent and less than 1 percent of the population was diabetic, it was 150 pounds. Oh, and the weight considered obese in 1911 for that five-foot-five woman was 171 pounds as opposed to 174 pounds today. What's up with that? Currently, there are studies underway that correlate being thinner with osteoporosis, that women who are heavier (though not obese) are less likely to develop osteoporosis. But the public is not barraged with information connecting thinness to any negative health effects. My point is that we can locate information about negative health effects of just about anything. So why does the media focus on one and not give attention to much else?

Because an idea is planted that will benefit the corporate structure: I am not good enough the way I am. How many times have you heard someone say, "I could stand to lose ten pounds," and inwardly agreed? We are programmed to think we need to be thinner and to admonish others for the way they look. We tell our children not to judge a book by its cover, and yet it is just that external criteria that media reinforces as supremely important. And this paves the way for all of the diet programs and weight-loss supplements. It is big business. And, as I said before, businesses don't care about personal health or happiness; they are only interested in their bottom line. Americans spend $35 billion a year on diet aids and $19.1 billion on gym memberships.[2] That's $54,100,000,000, which is more money than the state of New Jersey had in its proposed budget for 2013.[3]

This made me step back and think: our culture informs almost every aspect of our lives, whether we realize it or not. Television has become an integral part of American life. I enjoy TV, but I ask you to pay attention to the commercials. Fast food healthy meals? Lose weight by eating at a fast food joint? Even if you aren't "paying attention" to the ads, you are still getting the message. Your brain processes more information than you are aware that you are absorbing. This is called subliminal processing. So while you may not be "paying attention" to that "Flatter Abs in 6 Weeks" commercial, your brain is still digesting the information that you need flatter abs. Or that you can lose weight by eating at one fast food place over another. And because we equate weight loss with being healthier, we want to believe that nutritionally sound food is sold at a fast food store. We have a tendency not to pay attention to the language. Healthy and healthier are not the same words. A hoagie might be healthier than a hamburger, but are either really healthy?

There is no doubt that we as a society are getting less and less healthy. Food quality declines, overall health declines, and people start gaining weight, giving the "diet" industry a major boost. Diets work for a short time, and then people regain the weight, plus a little more, and the cycle starts all over again. This seems to be ignored. The media creates a focus on fat equaling unhealthy, not that increased body fat is a symptom created by the processed foods manufactured by the industrialized food system.

American perseverance when it comes to dieting is unparalleled. If one plan doesn't work, the dieter will move on to another. And when that one doesn't work, the perpetual dieter moves on again. The number of weight-loss programs and supplements seems to be growing exponentially. So with all of this dieting going on, why is it that Americans are getting fatter and fatter and less and less healthy? From 2000 to 2005, the prevalence of obesity increased by 24 percent. Interestingly, the numbers of the heaviest people (100–200 pounds overweight, for example) have increased the most. Obviously, something is amiss.

~~~~~~~

I'm not immune to this. I've gone on weight-loss diets. Plenty of them. Back in the late 1980s, my brother-in-law introduced my family to the Pritikin Diet. Nathan Pritikin purported that serious and life-threatening illnesses could be both caused by and treated with diet and exercise rather than conventional pharmaceutical methods. This wasn't exactly a new idea, but Dr. Pritikin had the chutzpah to battle with public and private health agencies, and even the American Medical Association, in an effort to change the way serious diseases were treated. Between 1976 and 1984, he developed an influential following, including medical doctors and scientists. I intimated earlier that there may be a link between contemporary eating habits and cancer rates; Dr. Pritikin boldly stated that he believed food to be both the poison and the antidote for the health problems plaguing America.[4] He wrote many books, including *The Pritikin Promise*, which I read from cover to cover. And going back to an old adage, if I am what I eat, then Nathan Pritikin's idea that diet could cure disease felt correct to me.

The Pritikin Promise was the first book I read that explained a rationale behind eating recommendations. It all seemed logical: less fat in, less fat on the body, less fat to clog up the works. I hadn't really studied anything about nutrition. I understood basic body chemistry: that the enzymes in saliva break down carbohydrates, the hydrochloric acid in the stomach breaks down proteins, and the enzyme/bacteria balance in the intestines takes care of the rest. However, my ideas about nutrition centered around this: whatever my mother told me was healthy was healthy.

By the mid 1990s, it seemed everyone was on the anti-fat band-wagon. Any food a body could crave became available in a non-fat form, from salad dressing to whipped cream. At the time, I remember feeling an inner conflict based upon what I read in Pritikin. On the upside, it was good that everything was fat-free. On the down-side, the food had tons of chemicals, which seemed to go against the whole-foods approach Pritikin took, and therefore went against what had originally made sense to me. I remember when Olean hit the market. I bought a bag of those chips, and man, did they make me sick! I had diarrhea for days, and only ate a few of them because I didn't think they tasted very good. I ate a low-fat diet for a few years, always struggling with my weight. I never thought about food trends; I never thought about my eating being fashionable. But that was all it was: the latest diet fashion.

And what of the myriad of other diet programs? They seem to contradict one another. I went back and reread Pritikin's theory before I started writing this chapter. I also read *Atkins for Life*, *The South Beach Diet*, and consulted WebMD about dieting and weight loss. I wanted to see what the authors of these programs had to say, not what the manufactured hype was doing in our market-driven economy. Surprisingly, these diets are not as far apart as they seem. Oh, they have pretty different ideas about fat/carbohydrate/protein ratios, but they all share three very important messages: replace refined grains with whole grains, avoid white sugar and other refined sweeteners (like high-fructose corn syrup), and eat a variety of nutrient-dense foods every day. This sounds oddly reminiscent of my grandmother's home economics textbook.

Every year, I have students "confess" to me that they didn't read one assigned book all year, as if I couldn't tell by the anemic responses they gave on their tests. They barely pass by talking to friends who read and looking things up on the internet. I see examples of this laziness in the larger culture, as well. I'll use Pritikin to illustrate my point. Most people won't bother reading exactly what Dr. Pritikin wrote because his writing style is dense. Most people will just listen to what someone else said, a sound bite on the local news perhaps, that excludes some very important information. For example, Dr. Pritikin wrote to "eat a lot of carbohydrates," but that wasn't the end of the sentence. He recommends eating a lot of carbohydrates *derived from whole foods*. Pritikin recommends whole-wheat pasta. Have you ever eaten whole-wheat pasta? The consistency is like damp cardboard, and it has a slightly sawdusty aftertaste. Okay, sure, it may be healthier, but I think it leaves a lot to be desired.

So how does the Pritikin Diet become so popular that it influences food industry marketing (the "low fat" and "fat free" monikers are effective product movers) if it recommends foods that have the consistency of something out of my recycling bin? The answer:

people take in only the part of the diet that is desirable and ignore the rest. Pritikin said high carbs, low fat. People think, "I like carbs," and start binge-eating refined, white-flour pasta. Twenty years of refined, white-flour pasta in large quantities. Look at what has happened to the American waistline in the past twenty years. Look at the waistline of the American child. What about the rise of gluten intolerance, celiac disease, and diabetes? Wouldn't the incredible increase in our consumption of refined carbohydrates directly correlate with a rise in these problems? The most frightening part for me is that people truly believe they are making food choices that will help them achieve maximum health when they choose refined pasta over a steak. Or that a bag of gummy candy is okay to eat because it is fat free. None of this is what Dr. Pritikin had in mind when he made his nutritional recommendations.

If we look past the 140-character interpretation of many popular diets, we find advice that parallels Grandma's wisdom and the tales of many old wives: eat real food that is full of nutrients. Notice I didn't use the word "healthy." "Healthy" has become a loaded word for advertisers. A food company can market a processed food as healthy if it is low in sodium and low in fat. Foods labeled "healthy" do not need to have any minimum level of nutritional value, just a sodium level of less than 140 milligrams per serving.

The human body needs sodium for many biological functions, and when we don't get salt in healthy ways, we crave it. When we crave, we look for the closest, easiest thing to satisfy that craving. When I was pregnant, I remember my OB telling me that if I was craving ice cream, I was probably really craving calcium and should eat a piece of cheese or drink some milk, which worked to satisfy the craving. Our bodies give us clues to what is lacking. The problem is that we no longer know how to listen to our bodies, nor how to fill the needs of our bodies. Ten years ago, approximately 30 percent of the population was hypertensive, and now with all of our lower sodium foods, that number has increased to 33 percent. All of this focus on individual ingredients, fat, and salt, and not a lot to show for it.

How to Make Fats a Friend

The food marketing industry's smear campaign on fats has almost completely managed to obscure the many uses and benefits of the substance. Animals come with fat. If you buy your meat straight from the farmer, you may find yourself scrambling for ways to use this oft-maligned substance. As you learn its many useful properties, you will learn that fats don't have to be an enemy.

Most fat straight from the animal has impurities that cause it to go rancid, so the fat gets rendered into things like tallow and lard to be used for cooking. We have used

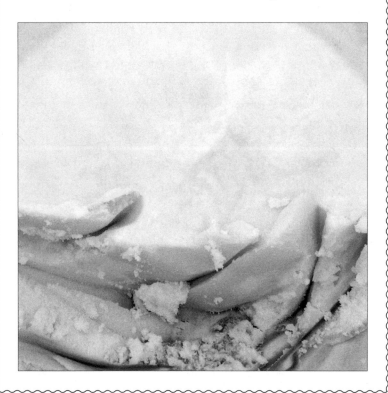

many rendering techniques, from boiling to slow cookers, but the best method I have come across is as follows.

Put the chunks of fat in an old colander and put the colander inside an oven-proof bowl. Put that on a baking sheet (to prevent disastrous spills) and place it in a 180°F oven until the fat melts. I have never scorched the fat using this method. Once the fat is rendered, strain it through a cheesecloth (or a piece of old cotton sheet—just be sure it is perfectly clean) to be sure there are not bits in it. Transfer the fat to freezer containers.

Lard (rendered pork fat) is my go-to fat. It's great for cooking because it adds a certain body to foods, but it doesn't really have a taste (despite its slight odor). It makes for the flakiest piecrust ever. I keep a container of my own piecrust mix in the freezer: combine 6 cups of flour with 1 teaspoon of baking powder and 1 tablespoon of salt. Cut in 1 pound of lard until it makes pebbles. For a two-crust pie, use 2 cups of mix combined with 1/3 cup of ice water. For a one-crust pie, use 1 cup of mix combined with 3 tablespoons of ice water.

I find tallow (rendered beef or mutton fat) a little strong for most cooking applications, so I use it for skin cream. It is an extremely effective defense for dry skin in the winter as well as skin irritations in the summer, including alleviating sunburn. Melt the tallow over a very low heat, just until there are no solids left, and remove it from the heat. For every cup of tallow, add 2 tablespoons of extra virgin olive oil to make it spreadable. I also add essential oils to improve the smell—peppermint, lavender, and sage are particularly effective for covering the meaty odor. This mixture can also make a nice lip balm if you add orange oil.

Recently, the *American Journal of Clinical Nutrition* published a meta-analysis of twenty-one studies that concluded the "intake of saturated fats was not associated with an increased risk of coronary heart disease, stroke, or cardiovascular disease."[5] Recent research has stressed the importance of fats for brain development and better memory. Why weren't these findings more widely publicized? Consider the economic impact if people suddenly stopped buying and consuming refined foods (the real culprit) and stopped having heart attacks. The diet industry and the industrial food system would suffer.

Part of why fat became such an easy target in the diet wars is because that is exactly what we are trying to remove from our bodies—pounds of "ugly fat." This cultural obsession with fat removal, with thinness, drives gazillions of people to jump on the current diet bandwagon and buy into it. I don't care if it is Weight Watchers, Pritikin, or a marketing-savvy fast food joint; as soon as someone loses weight and keeps it off for six months, everyone who has not succeeded in doing the same jumps on that train and tries to ride it. However, if you read the fine print at the bottom of the ad, you'll see that "Results are not typical." Fads do not work; they lack balance.

Obesity is a symptom of our irrational approach to food. Rather than looking for the sources that create symptoms, we tend to just alleviate symptoms. A symptom is a physical manifestation that alerts us that something is wrong. A runny nose and a fever are symptoms of infection, and they are indicators that let us know the body is fighting the infection. The runny nose is not the problem. The fever is not the problem. While the symptoms may be annoying or even dangerous, just getting the nose to stop running and the fever to go away does not mean the infection has cleared up. People take antibiotics to fight the infection, and continue taking the antibiotics for days after the symptoms have cleared because even though the symptoms have gone away, the infection may still be in the body. I see obesity like that runny nose and fever—it is a symptom that something is wrong with the body. It could be the way the body is fueled, a hormone malfunction, or even a spiritual or emotional trauma. But rather than searching out a cause, the first thing most people do is go on a diet; they try to alleviate the symptom, not fix the problem. And by diet, I mean that they implement some type of dietary restriction intended for weight loss. Sometimes people are successful in losing the weight and keeping it off. To me, this means that those people changed the way they perceive and use food. But because of the tendency to alleviate the symptom (being overweight) rather than finding a cause, many people suffer from weight yo-yoism. They lose fifty pounds and then gain it all back, and sometimes more. Why the high failure rate? Because we aren't learning truly healthier, balanced ways to eat. We focus and obsess on the restrictions. We eat the processed food provided by the program, lose weight, and then go back to regular processed food and gain it all back again.

~~~~~~~~

I remember, when I was a kid, eating a huge Jersey white peach and my mom sticking a bowl under it because I had already soaked through two napkins and was making a huge mess all over the kitchen table. I look at the peaches in a local orchard and understand that they aren't as big as the ones I remember because I've grown (and everything looks smaller, eh?), but they are still really juicy and make a huge mess when eaten (I send my kids outside). So what is so important about that drippy peach? When that peach reached its full ripeness, all of its vitamins and minerals reached their peak potency. This is true for all fruits and vegetables. The quality of the usable vitamins and minerals improves as the food ripens. Once again, a commonsense observation: our bodies are programmed to desire the foods that are best for us. So "sweet" was not always an enemy. Once upon a time, developed sugars in fruits and vegetables were Nature's way of telling us that the fruit or vegetable was ready to be eaten.

Once mankind began refining sugar and it became readily available, we added it to foods during processing and as a form of preservation (turning fruit into jam, for example), and health-wise things began to go downhill. Dr. Weston Price did extensive research back in the 1930s and wrote an in-depth, profound tome chronicling his research called *Nutrition and Physical Degeneration*. Dr. Price studied cultures from around the globe, comparing groups of indigenous peoples, some of whom followed a diet that was traditional for the regions with others who had adopted a Western diet (the precursor of the Standard American Diet [SAD] that makes use of refined flour and sugar). In culture after culture, Dr. Price found that those groups who followed their traditional diets were in markedly better health than those who had adopted the diet of white flour, sugar, and processed foods.[6] The timing of this research was critical because there were still pockets of cultures that had not adopted a Westernized diet of refined foods. It would be difficult at best to duplicate Dr. Price's studies today.

The refining process varies, but most foods begin as a whole unit. I'll use grain as an example. A whole grain is a seed, and Nature, being a truly amazing and wondrous keeper, creates a unit of food that has the correct proportion of nutrients in order for the body to make the most of them, when properly prepared. Therefore, when a whole grain is eaten, the person is eating a unit of food that has all of its complementary nutritional values: enough vitamins to use the protein and enough vitamins to complement the fiber, and so on. Most of the diets I researched promote eating whole grains because a whole grain is a better nutritional choice than a refined grain. Whole grains naturally have vitamin E, a boatload of B vitamins, and minerals that are essential to good health. The refining process strips the vitamins along with the fiber. In order to return some nutritional value to the product, manufacturers fortify the product with synthetic vitamins and minerals. The fortification cannot match the exact balance of nutrients that were in the grain at the beginning and therefore the refined product is less healthy.

In addition, naturally occurring vitamins and minerals are more easily absorbed by the body than synthetic vitamins.

Back to Pritikin and his use of whole grains. There are recipes in the book, because at the time it was published there was no Pritikin food line. He suggested homemade foods because there was no place to go out and buy Pritikin food. He was a man, not a brand. Nowhere in *The Pritikin Promise* is there a hint that anyone should be eating processed foods. Nowadays, Pritikin has its own line of pre-packaged foods that include whole grains. And guess what? Both Atkins and South Beach also recommend whole food, and each of these programs now includes an entire line of processed foods—just what the original texts say to avoid. Amazing what happens when capitalist interests overtake health interests.

I find myself at a basic commonsense question: what is the point of taking all of these nutrients out of the product just to put them back in? Most might say, "Because it tastes better." White flour doesn't really have a flavor. Freshly ground whole-wheat flour has a pleasant nutty flavor. Many people do not like whole-wheat products, objecting on the grounds that whole-wheat products don't taste as good as white flour products. Usually it isn't flavor at all, but texture: how the food product feels in the mouth. Thanks to the myriad of refining processes and the fast food industry, Americans have become Goldilocks, expecting food to have a certain texture—not too chewy, not too mushy, not too crunchy, and definitely not grainy. Therefore, foods are processed for better texture or mouth-feel.

Like I said, I am not going to tell you what to eat or how to lose weight, because that isn't the object of this book. I just want to share what I have learned over the past ten years. The best nutritional advice I have ever heard is the last common element in the diets I read: eat a balance of nutrient-dense foods. What is a nutrient-dense food? A whole food. A complete unit, created in nature with its own balanced array of nutrients, like an egg. You may worry about the cholesterol, but an egg is a unit of food, packed in its own protective coating, with the right amount of fat and vitamin E to make its protein available for use. Everything is about balance.

NOTES

[1] Ideal Weight Calculator, Calculator.Net, http://www.calculator.net/ideal-weight -calculator.html (accessed November 2014).

[2] Melissa McNamara, "Diet Industry is Big Business," CBSnews.com, February 11, 2009 (accessed January 2013); Keith Cronin, "Investing in Exercise," *Suite 101*, February 25, 2010 (accessed July 2010).

[3] Chris Christie, "Governor's FY 2013 Budget," New Jersey State, Office of Management and Budget, 2012, http://www.state nj.us/treasury/omb.

[4] Tom Monte, "All About Pritikin," Pritikin Longevity Center, July 7, 2010, http://www.pritikin.com/index.php?option=com_content&view=article&id=61&Item id=89.

[5] Patty Siri-Tarino and Qi Sun, "Meta-analysis of Prospective Cohort Studies Evaluating the Association of Saturated Fat with Cardiovascular Disease," *American Journal of Clinical Nutrition* 91, 3 (July 2010): www.ajcn.org/cgi/content/abstract/91/3/535.

[6] Weston Price, *Nutrition and Physical Degeneration* (LaMesa, CA: The Price-Pottenger Nutritional Foundation, 1939).

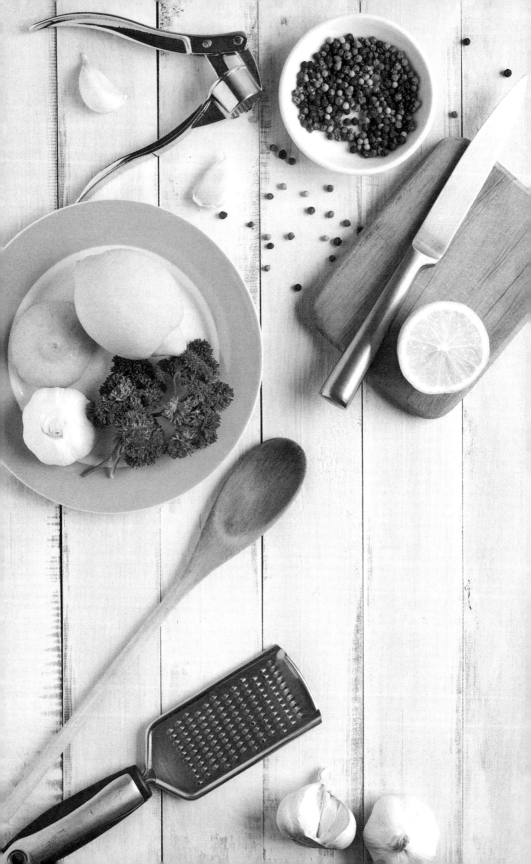

The Food Maze

SEEING THE BOUNDARIES

3

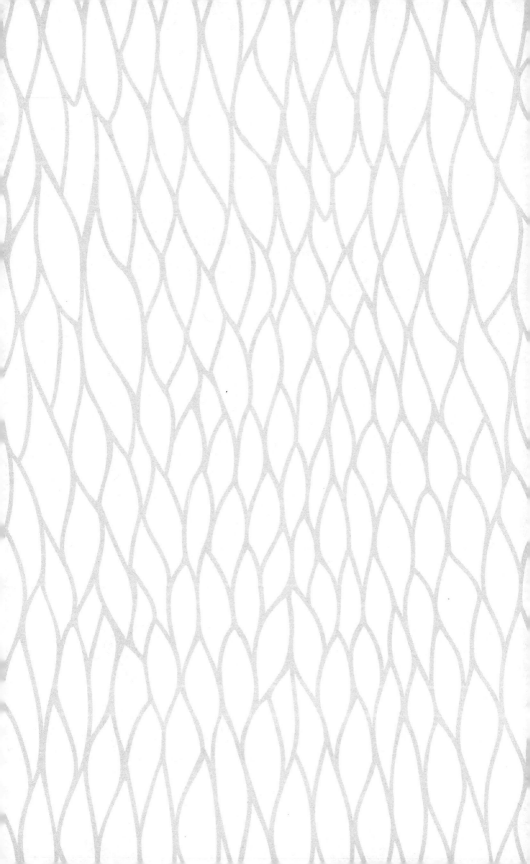

I t's an all-too-common refrain nowadays: "I wish I had the time, but I'm too busy!" Home-cooked meals and family dinners have, of apparent necessity, taken a backseat to the never-ending busy-work of contemporary life. In a world of modern conveniences and time-saving technology that would've been un-imaginable less than a century ago, how is that we now have less time to prepare food for our families?

In order to understand how Americans have gotten so busy, we must consider the twenty-first-century American lifestyle and how it is affected by the distorted reflection of the ever-present media. According to a 2014 Nielsen report, the average American between the ages of thirty-five and forty-nine watches over thirty-three hours of television per week.[1] We are bombarded by images of a super-mom who works outside the home at a job that allows her to attend every event in her children's lives. She is her daughter's BFF but maintains parental authority. Her house is clean, her laundry done, and her yard as manicured as her hands because her husband (with whom she never argues) helps her with everything. Commercial Dad is never angry; he drives his children to school in a racecar and provides well-balanced breakfasts for his family; there is always time to play catch with Son and soothe Daughter's heartaches. The children are clean, conservatively dressed, and well-adjusted. In comparison, how can we not feel like failures? Even supposed middle-class families on television are not presented in a middle-class context. Think about the backdrop: how big is that house? That yard? Would the granite countertops in the kitchen be worth half of the fictional family's annual income?

A study by independent market research company Ipsos Open Exchange found that the average adult spends well over two hours per day using social media.[2] How much of your precious spare time is spent looking through other people's vacation photos, children's achievements, and decorating plans? With the constant easy access to social media, it's hard to keep in mind that you're only seeing the best and brightest moments that people have chosen to share of their lives; no one's true life experience would fit pleasantly on a Pinterest board. Remember, comparison is the thief of joy.

Studies have shown a correlation between increased media consumption and a distorted view of affluence in the real world. In a 1997 study, participants were asked how common it was to own certain luxury items, like hot tubs or convertibles. Presumably because they'd frequently seen these things on television, participants who were heavy television viewers overestimated how prevalent these items actually were. Researchers concluded, "'Knowing' how others live informs consumer expectations, satisfaction, motivation, and desire.... Representations of social reality frame and situate human behavior, including consumer behavior."[3] If all your favorite television families employ live-in maids on their middle-class salaries, you may begin to wonder why you can't afford to do so, too.

Many people find themselves in debt up to their eyeballs trying to keep up with these images of how their lives should be as presented in these fictional worlds, so they work more hours to pay the bills. Social media–savvy parents of children involved in sports may feel peer-pressured into buying special cleats, arranging private training sessions, and scheduling nutritional consultations so that their child can measure up to his peers. We don't want to be considered miserly, so we contribute generously to our churches, synagogues, and charities, and we volunteer on the PTA. We work very hard and spend a lot of time and effort trying to reconcile who we are with the image the media presents of who we "should" be.

The disparity between who we really are and who we think we need to be is good for convenience food, fast food, and the corporate food model. As we struggle to keep up with the media image of who we are supposed to be, the less time we perceive that we have, the less time we will spend cooking food for ourselves, even if the activities keeping us busy are ostensibly meant to keep us healthy as well. My friend once told me, "I was so tired after I got done at the gym, I just stopped at McDonald's and got burgers for my family." I never teach the concept of doublethink in George Orwell's *1984* without thinking of that line.

It is important to be aware of how many variables other than food itself influence what, why, and how we eat. And what we eat influences who we are. We can't listen to our bodies anymore because we have become addicted to additives and refined foods. So I am back to checking in with Grandma. Not that "clean your plate" business—that's part of the problem. We grew up being told to clean our plates, but we no longer cook whole foods or eat single servings. We eat at restaurants that provide portions large enough to feed two people, from food that has compromised nutritional value.

Ask Grandma where food came from seventy years ago. She'd mention the green grocer, the butcher, the fishmonger, and the milkman who delivered milk from cows on nearby farms. Now grocery shopping is centralized: we go to the grocery store and get everything we need. The milk we drink might come from ten different dairies, and when it gets to the distributor, it all gets mixed together. From the distributor it gets bottled and shipped anywhere in the country. Milk from New Jersey might end up in Ohio! This centralization in the food industry, on many levels, reflects our cultural expectations: everything needs to be convenient and should taste "the same." So while Grandma spent the day in and out of stores getting all of her grocery needs for the next couple of days, we chauffeur children hither and yon and stop at the CVS to grab a couple of frozen pizzas and a twelve-pack of sodas to consume while we finish crunching some numbers for work.

It's as if our entire culture has slipped into a corporate model, trying to hold us accountable to a time clock we've forgotten we can control. We adults are the ones who sign our children up for three clubs and sixteen sports teams and then complain about all of the running around and chauffeuring and how little time we have. As I said in chapter 1, we are busy at our jobs, but very few of us are employed in situations where we can physically see what we did in a given day. We don't have the cabinet that we built in front of us; we don't have baskets of apples we picked in the cold cellar. Without visual affirmation of accomplishment for the day, we create exhaustion for ourselves to feel as though we have accomplished something.

One of the many downsides of our fast food culture is that food is no longer a revered cultural icon. This is probably one of the most detrimental aspects of our diet: the myriad of fast food restaurants are cultural icons and Sunday dinner with the family is not.

When did the family meal become an event that occurs twice or three times a year, for major holidays? One of the easiest ways to connect or reconnect with your family is over a meal, yet the family meal is often forgotten or dismissed as "old-fashioned" and, therefore, unnecessary. Studies conducted by the American Psychological Association, the National Center on Addiction and Substance Abuse, and various major universities support the assertion that there is a direct correlation between frequent family meals and children who are less likely to use illegal drugs, drink alcohol, and be sexually promiscuous.[4] In addition, these children usually have better success in school, higher self-esteem, fewer problems with depression, and a lower incidence of obesity.[5]

I will suggest that you stop for a moment and ask yourself what is most important to you. If you picked up this book, then nutrition and food are things that are important to you; sorting out this maze, or labyrinth, of information, disinformation, and misinformation about food is important to you. What you are willing to take out of your schedule in order to improve the health and welfare of your family?

Putting Snacks in your Corner

The urge to snack on something fast and convenient can lure even the most resolute traveler off the path to food empowerment. If you're looking to make a lasting change to your eating habits, it's best to start slowly. Avoid temptation by keeping healthy, easy-to-make foods on hand. Try replacing store-bought yogurt with homemade for a healthy family snack.

HOMEMADE GREEK–STYLE YOGURT

3 1/2 cups of whole milk (see note)
1/2 cup plain yogurt (either commercial with live cultures
    or reserved from your last batch)
candy thermometer

Heat the milk on the stove slowly. If you are using **pasteurized** milk, heat to 180°F and let cool to 110°F. If you are using **raw** milk, heat to 110°F. Whisk in the 1/2 cup yogurt. Transfer to a quart-size mason jar and place the jar and a heating pad inside a little cooler. Turn the heating pad to medium. Incubate for 4–8 hours, depending on how tart you like your yogurt. The longer it sits, the more tart it will be. After the yogurt has incubated, put it in the refrigerator until it is completely cooled (I usually leave it overnight). The next morning, place a flour sack towel inside a sieve and place the sieve on a bowl. If you have used raw milk, scrape the "cream" from the top and reserve in a small bowl. Put the rest of the yogurt in the sieve. Put it back in the fridge and let it strain for about an hour. Reserve the whey, the yellowish liquid, for lacto-fermenting (see chapter 4 and appendix B for more on using whey); it will keep in a jar in the fridge for a couple of months. Invert the sieve into the bowl and peel the towel off the yogurt and whisk the "cream" back into the yogurt and enjoy! My children love this yogurt salted for dipping vegetables.

Note: I feel that grass-fed raw milk gives the best, most consistent results. If you cannot get raw milk, try to find grass-fed milk that is not homogenized. If you can't find that, then settle for organic milk that has not been ultra-pasteurized.

How much time do you spend watching television each week, or browsing Facebook or Pinterest, or playing video games? I bet it's more than you think. My friends admit to an average of twenty-four hours of TV a week, plus two or three hours on Facebook, unless they are playing the games, which would up them to ten hours a week. I had one friend tell me that she could lose an entire afternoon surfing Pinterest. And yet they say it's impossible to find three or four hours a week to put meals together. It isn't that difficult to prep out four or five meals at once on a Sunday afternoon and save yourself a lot of time during the week. In addition to keeping you out of restaurants and away from the take-out menu, preparing meals creates an opportunity for a family bonding activity with a sense of purpose.

Another downside to the Everything Fast posture that we've adopted is that it leads us to want instant change and instant results. You can't expect your family to sit down to dinner every night after years of not doing so. You can't expect that you will suddenly have the energy and inspiration to cook dinner every night if you really don't know how to cook. My personal journey took place over ten years—a decade of small steps that led us to where we are now. Diet programs designed to get a dieter off to a quick start have been very popular and successful in the short-term, but how many people actually keep that weight off? Habits are hard to break, and the American mind-set about food is a habit, a habit that we need to change.

Focus on one step at a time, slow down, and take the time to really incorporate one small change, and you can make it stick. My son now puts his dirty clothes in the hamper. It took months of daily reminders. He had no other new chore, just getting his dirty clothes in the hamper. Is he perfect with this chore? Of course not. I still find sock-balls under his bed on occasion (or in the couch cushions), but most of the time, his dirty clothes are in the hamper, which is a major improvement over finding his dirty clothes on the floor wherever he happened to get changed. We can't expect perfection, but that shouldn't stop us from striving toward it.

Will this take effort? Yes. However, I am an average working-outside-the-home mom and I have gained control over my food. You have a lot more control over your food than you think, as well. Your commitment level is up to you, and it will wax and wane. The most important thing is to stay honest with yourself. Know your limits. And in this case, don't have expectations of any immediate, complete permanent change. Make decisions one at a time, so that they will be decisions with which you can live.

NOTES

[1] David Hinckley, "Average American Watches 5 Hours of TV Per Day, Report Shows," *New York Daily News*, March 5, 2014, http://www.nydailynews.com/life-style/average-american-watches-5-hours-tv-day-article-1.1711954.

[2] "Socialogue: The Most Common Butterfly on Earth Is the Social Butterfly," Ipsos, January 8, 2013, http://ipsos-na.com/news-polls/pressrelease.aspx?id=5954.

[3] Thomas O'Guinn and L. J. Shrum, "The Role of Television in the Construction of Consumer Reality," *Journal of Consumer Research*, 23 (March 1997): 278–94, http://www.e-campus.uvsq.fr/claroline/backends/download.php?url=L0FydGljbGVzL08tJ0d1aW5fU2hydW1fMTk5N19KQ1IucGRm&cidReset=true&cidReq=CL.

[4] "The Importance of Family Dinners VII," CASAColumbia, September 2012, http://www.casacolumbia.org/addiction-research/reports/importance-of-family-dinners-2012.

[5] Lindsay A. Schwarz, "Effects of Family Mealtime Practices on Household Inhabitants," Eastern Illinois University *Undergraduate Research Journal for the Human Sciences* 4 (2005): http://www.kon.org/urc/v4/schwarz.html; "The Importance of Family Dinners," University of Florida Institute of Food and Agricultural Sciences Extension, http://solutionsforyourlife.ufl.edu/hot_topics/families_and_consumers/family_dinners.html (accessed August 2014).

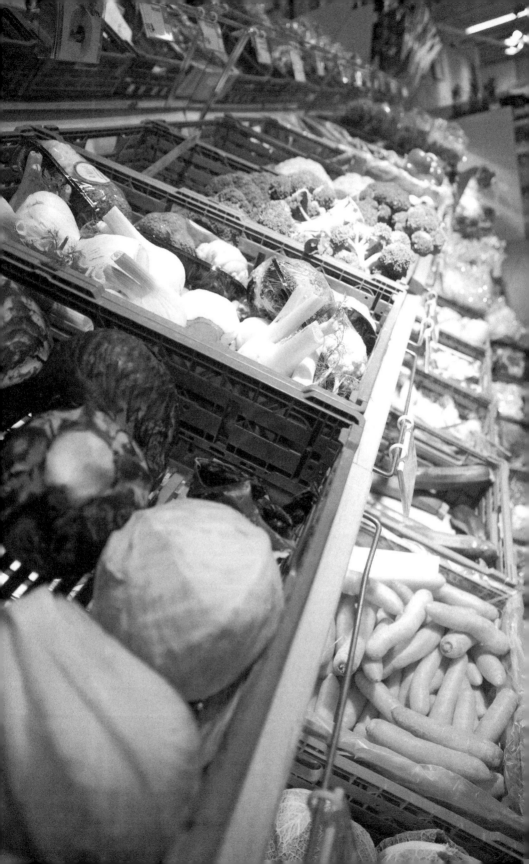

CORPORATE MARKETING MANIPULATION

CONTEXT CREATES STORY

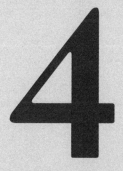

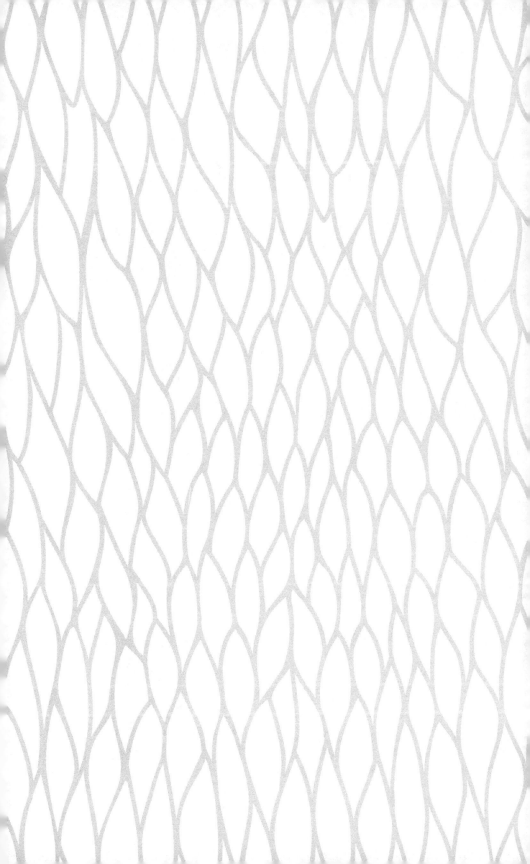

Everyone has an agenda. Food companies want you to buy their food, so they pay big money for research and development of new more convenient foods for you to consume, with lots of fancy packaging for you to throw away (or recycle). They pay for advertising campaigns, and they convince you that you need their products, maybe through fear (I won't have enough time unless I use this—panic, panic), maybe through insecurity (all the cool moms give their kid this), or maybe through status (it's the best money can buy). I have an agenda, as well: You don't need what Industrial Food is trying to sell you. As a matter of fact, what Industrial Food is trying to sell you might be the exact opposite of what you need.

Financial Context

Money influences almost every aspect of the American culture. Don't think for a minute that some corporate mogul doesn't drive our nutritional information. Corporations are involved with the government through lobby interests and campaign contributions. Fundamentally it is one of the rudimentary principles of the American Dream: if I work hard, I will be prosperous. We have a separation of church and state in this country, but we do not have a separation of government and capitalism. They work hand-in-hand, and to think that FDA or USDA recommendations are not influenced by corporate interests is just naive.

Political Context

The CEO of a food corporation is no different from the CEO of a munitions corporation. The CEO runs the company and is responsible to a board of directors who expects the company to turn a profit. Anonymous Food Corporation contributes money to a certain PAC group that endorses Candidate Herbert. Herbert gets elected on the campaign promise of a chicken finger in every microwave, goes to Washington, and votes to pass legislation that subsidizes farmers who grow chickens. The subsidy lowers the cost of production of chickens, so that when Anonymous Food Corporation purchases the harvest, the financial output is minimal. Anonymous Food Corporation processes the chicken into hundreds of different food-stuffs, sold all across the country. Anonymous Food Corporation makes a huge profit. In order to save some tax money, the Anonymous Food Corporation contributes to a parallel charitable fund that works alongside the PAC to which they contributed last year. The charitable fund does work for the PAC that alleviates an area that would have cost the PAC money. The PAC endorses a candidate, and there are chicken fingers in every microwave.

Nutritional Context

In order for this process to be effective, corporations need consumers to purchase their goods. Therefore, our diet is contextually influenced by an industrialized corporate food system that plays to a public manipulated by advertising. American consumption of refined flour, refined sugar, refined corn (such as high-fructose corn syrup or corn oil), and refined soy (such as a protein supplement, preservative, or oil) has gone up astronomically. It is estimated that Americans eat a diet that is 80 percent white flour, sugar, and oil.[1] Adult obesity is a growing problem (pardon the pun). The incidence of cancer is going up at a parabolic rate. The number of people with diabetes is going up. Attention deficit disorder (ADD) and attention deficit hyperactivity disorder (ADHD) are affecting more and more children. The number of people affected by allergies and asthma is going up. Autism and Asperger's are on the rise, and of course, there's an epidemic of childhood obesity. Our collective health is worsening, and people are starting to see a correlation. The mass food supply has become nutritionally void. Why has no action been taken to change the food supply?

If we are not fueling our bodies with nutrient-dense foods, our bodies will move into a state of decline. The solution is simple: buy nutrient-dense food. Implementation of the solution is not so simple. If white flour, sugar, and oil make up 80 percent of the standard American diet, then that is what will take up most of the food market. First of all, the processed food industry has more money coming into its coffers, which means it has more money to spend on advertising. Second, look at your grocery store—fresh food around the perimeter, and processed foods up and down the aisles: Oh no, not geometry! That's right: Area takes up more of the store than the perimeter.

Purchasing Context

Every building design has a purpose, and grocery stores are no different. Many factors are taken into consideration, from energy efficiency to creating counterclockwise traffic flow for better sales. Did you ever notice that most grocery stores entrances are at the fresh produce section, usually on the right-hand side of the store? Why? Because fresh produce is pretty. It's bright and colorful and makes a positive psychological impact that you will carry with you on your counterclockwise odyssey through the space. Milk and eggs are placed in the opposite corner from the produce, which draws you through the store. From the moment you enter the store, you are being manipulated to buy.

In terms of packing your shopping cart, why would you begin with produce? It's some of the most fragile food you buy, so it would make sense for it to be near the end of the shopping trip to be on the top of the cart—on top of the frozen items, so it would stay cool while you wait in the checkout line. Stores start you off in the produce section to instill a sense of freshness. For example, the lettuce looks as if it just came in from the field, covered with morning dew. Fat chance, especially if it's December and you live in Wisconsin. It may have traveled two thousand miles over a week or so. But with the wilted exterior leaves removed, and misted by the spray nozzles mounted on the produce open merchandiser, their appearance makes many consumers confident they are choosing the freshest lettuce ever.

There has been quite a bit of media about shopping around the perimeter of the grocery store because that is where the items that give the most nutrition per calorie usually can be found. One of the economic issues is that the items around the edges tend to be more expensive than those on the interior. A bag of chips is less expensive than four apples. A box of store-brand macaroni and cheese is a lot cheaper than a wedge of cheese from the dairy case. This has to do with government subsidies to certain foods, as well as the relative costs of manufacturing. That box of mac-n-cheese has a long shelf life. The wedge of cheese doesn't. Therefore, the box is less expensive to have in the store because it doesn't have that short time period of viability for sale that the wedge of cheese does. In the long run, however, if macaroni and cheese is a staple of my diet, and I factor in the medical costs for potential problems like obesity or vitamin costs to supplement the missing nutrients, I might find that the wedge of cheese is a better buy. On the other hand, if I am on a limited food budget, I am going to purchase what I can afford. Why would I spend $5.98 on a chunk of cheese when for two cents more I could buy twenty-four boxes of store-brand macaroni and cheese when it goes on sale?

Store layout is not the only way businesses influence consumers when it comes to grocery shopping. Shopping has a great deal of loaded, trigger vocabulary. Splashy logos proclaiming "50% less!" make people stop to look, and maybe consider putting the item into the cart. But 50 percent less of what? A bag of low-fat potato chips could contain more carbohydrates than the original variety. The phrase "new low-sodium recipe" is meant to trigger an association with "healthier," but unless you're hypertensive, the low-sodium recipe may not be the healthier option for you. Language, the vocabulary of food, can be deceptive. Language that concerns food is constantly changing, and the fact that some of the language is regulated and some of the language is not creates a situation where the consumer is very apt to be misled by food manufacturers. Words can change meaning when they change context.

Let's start with a key word concerning a growing marketing niche: organic. When it comes to food, "organic" is a regulated term with very specific meaning. But first let's consider the connotation of the word.

When most people think about organics, they think beans, rice, and things that take forever to prepare and/or cost a lot to buy. If I ask you to close your eyes and visualize someone who eats organic food, you might picture a latter-day hippie snacking on granola behind the wheel of a VW bus; or maybe a yuppie mom in a yoga outfit, just looking for something on which to spend her ample free time and disposable income; or maybe even the crazy English teacher you had in high school. You might picture the person sauntering up and down the aisles of some swanky market, gently placing items in a basket and then packing those items into reusable bags at the checkout. Okay, I am an English teacher, and I do have reusable grocery bags, but I'm more of a toss-it-in-the-cart and run-down-the next-aisle kind of shopper, narrowly avoiding the guy who I think is a whack job but is really just talking into a Bluetooth. People who eat organic food are just regular people. So why do they do it? And what makes organic food organic?

Organic does not mean vegetarian. Organic is not a trendy marketing tool or a snobby status marker (at least, it wasn't originally). Organic is a dynamic term. Things that are organic come about naturally, not according to a societal standard or timetable; not according to profit margins or demands of the market. For example, my family and I came to our current eating style through organic means. We did not wake up one day and decide to change overnight. One change grew naturally out of the changes that preceded it over the course of the past ten years.

How does this apply to food? Organic food is produced without the use of synthetic chemicals, synthetic pesticides, antibiotics and/or hormones (either by injection or through the feed). As more and more evidence is uncovered linking pesticides and chemical additives to maladies like ADD/ADHD, autism, and higher incidences of cancer, the demand for organic foods is growing. This increase in demand is pushing organic food from a small niche market to big business.[2]

One needs to know the difference between all-natural and organic. These terms are not used interchangeably. An apple, picked from a local orchard, is all-natural. The apple is a fruit, produced by the flower of the tree that was pollinated, a natural process. However, if that apple had a chemical applied to it to keep the bugs away (a.k.a. a chemical pesticide), then that apple is not organic. It may be the tastiest apple you ever put in your mouth, but I'd advise you to wash it first. In order for an item to be all-natural, it must be naturally produced and not chemically converted. The FDA does not regulate the term "all-natural," and there is a movement for manufacturers to stop using it because of its potential to mislead consumers. Obviously, all-natural is not representative of the same standard as organic. The "Certified Organic" label is used only on items produced within strict and very specific regulations. In addition, the product and producer must be inspected and approved by an accredited certifying agent. "The USDA Federal Rule governing organic certification requires that an organic production system is managed to respond to site-specific conditions by integrating cultural, biological, and mechanical practices that foster cycling of resources, promote ecological balance, and conserve biodiversity."[3] If you are unsure, check the packaging. Only organic products should carry an organic label.

I do not want to go into a long explanation of monoculture, polyculture, and biodiversity here, but in order to understand another big deal in food labels, "GMO-Free," a brief explanation of these terms is necessary. A monoculture is a farm that cultivates one crop, generally one of two crops that are sometimes alternated from year to year, usually corn and soybeans. Polyculture refers to a farm that uses biodiversity by planting many varieties of crops on the same plot of land. There are numerous environmental and economic issues with monoculture farming, including the crop's increased vulnerability to pests and diseases. Monoculture crops are generally genetically similar strains developed for yield. When a pest or disease comes along that devastates that variety, the entire crop could be wiped out (think the Great Irish Potato Famine). Conventional (nonorganic) farmers are planting fewer and fewer varieties of plants. How are they avoiding pest problems? Through biotechnology, particularly gene modification, in which DNA is transferred from one organism to another. The transferred DNA changes the characteristics of the receiving organism,[4] thus creating a genetically modified organism, or GMO.

There has been a lot of controversy lately over whether or not GMO food products should be labeled in the United States. A few states have voted on legislation to require all GMO products to bear labels, and biotech companies like Monsanto have spent millions trying to oppose these measures. Why all the fuss? This new technology has been used to produce plants that resist herbicides, that don't mind crowding, that are resistant to certain pests and diseases. These are useful results, so what's the problem? We have no idea what effect these genetically modified organisms might have on our health and well-being. Look at high-fructose corn syrup, once thought to be a cheap, innocuous alternative to sugar, now suspected to be a major contributor to the obesity epidemic and some liver problems. Nearly ten years ago, Dr. Meira Field was doing research on the effect of HFCS on lab rats. While glucose can be metabolized by all cells, fructose is only metabolized in the liver. "The livers of the rats on the high fructose diet looked like the livers of alcoholics, plugged with fat and cirrhotic."[5] GMOs have only been on the commercial market since 1994. So far no studies have definitively linked GMOs with health problems, but the nature of genetics is complicated, and it's impossible to know what further study will reveal. What harm could GM food create? I have no clue, but I sure don't want my children to be the lab rats for the effects of GM foods. I guess, in a sense, I am volunteering them for the control group.

Most commercial GMO crops have been engineered to be resistant to glyphosate-based pesticides, meaning that when the farmers spray a field with glyphosates, all pests and weeds die, but the crop survives. This resistance is touted as lowering the number and toxicity of pesticides needed for monoculture crops. Unfortunately, after frequent use, weeds and pests develop a resistance to glyphosate, leading the farmer to spray more and more pesticides. The widespread use of GMO crops is actually increasing the number of toxic pesticides sprayed into our environment.[6]

What if genetically modified pollen lands on non-genetically modified stamens? The resulting produce from the non-GMO pollinated by the GMO exhibits GMO traits. Therefore, a farmer who did not wish to grow GMO foods is suddenly, and without his knowledge or consent, growing GMOs! Although the rules for organic crops forbid the use of GMOs, natural cross-pollination between GMO and organic crops—for example if the wind blows pollen from GMO soy to an organic farm's soy—does not count as usage. It is entirely possible for organic crops to contain small amounts of GMO material.[7] GMOs are already everywhere. I went to find information to estimate the percentage of crops that are GMO crops and found very conflicting numbers. Some sources report that over 90 percent of soy and 70 percent of corn planted worldwide are genetically modified.

～～～

When we discuss processed food, what does "processed" mean? In a sense, we process just about everything. Having an animal slaughtered and butchered is processing. Making pickles is processing. Cooking is a form of processing. But when we use the word "processed" in terms of contemporary food, we mean refined food created in a factory. Food created in factories relies on preservatives to help the food stay fresh, and plenty of salt and sugar (or, more likely, high-fructose corn syrup because it is less expensive) to make them taste good. What is the effect of all of this processed food?

Lacto-Fermentation
FAST AND EASY PRESERVATION

Lacto-fermentation is probably one of the oldest forms of preservation, likely preceding even oral history. As soon as someone figured out that the cabbage that got splashed with sea water tasted good for a long time after most cabbage had become a moldy mess, lacto-fermentation was practiced! No matter which corner of the world you choose, if you look into the culinary history, you will find a form of fermentation.

Lacto-fermentation preserves food using lactobacilli, one of the good-for-your-gut bacteria, to convert sugars and starches into lactic acid, creating a pH that prevents bad bacteria from growing on the food. Interestingly, bacteria that are potentially dangerous to our digestive systems cannot tolerate salt, so the preserved food is either salted or submerged in a salt brine to prevent the growth of harmful bacteria. Lactobacilli are salt tolerant and survive this first stage of the process. Then begins fermentation. The fermentation process will produce air bubbles in the jar. If you make pickles or other brined whole vegetables, you might see the spices floating up and then dropping down to the bottom.

In addition to preserving the food, the process of lacto-fermentation changes the chemical structure of the food so that it is actually more nutritious. It delivers more vitamins to the body and an abundance of good flora to the intestines.

My own interest in lacto-fermentation was sparked by the question of what to do with the whey I had leftover from straining yogurt. The writings of Sally Fallon and Sandor Ellix Katz only furthered my interest. If you worry that you won't like the flavor of lacto-fermented foods, start by eating them "young," when they have just finished the initial fermentation. The foods are less sour. I was not really much of a sauerkraut fan before I started making my own kraut.

Lacto-fermentation requires the use of salt. I recommend unrefined sea salt, for the most nutrition. If you want to cut back on the salt, you can use whey as a dairy-based bacterial "starter culture" to get the fermentation going. While you can purchase whey from many sources on the web, it is very easy to make your own whey as a by-product of making homemade Greek-style yogurt (see recipe in chapter 3).

General Lacto-Fermenting Instructions

For vegetable fermentation, you can use any glass jar that has a tight-fitting lid and is thoroughly cleaned. I generally use wide-mouth canning jars because that is what I have on hand. I prefer the plastic lids to the metal lids that are included with the jars. Some mayonnaise lids fit the wide mouth jars, but you must be sure that it is a tight fit!

Pack the jars tightly, making sure that the tops of the vegetables are covered by the liquid, whether it be exuded from the vegetables from being salted or the brine used to cover. Be sure to leave at least an inch of space (called head room) between the vegetables and the top of the jar. Leave the jars in a warm spot for two to three days. The second stage of fermentation is where the formation of the good-for-your-gut bacteria happens. The longer you leave ferments on the counter, the more bacteria will form, so check on them regularly. When you see that lots of bubbles have formed, the jars are ready to transfer to cold storage. Our house does not have air conditioning, so sometimes in the summer months, I have put ferments into cold storage after as little as thirty-six hours. In the fall when I am making kraut, I have had jars on the counter for up to two weeks. The bubbles are the key. Also, you must use filtered water or well water—water that has not been chlorinated. Chlorination inhibits the growth of the lactobacilli.

Cold storage means a cold place where the temperatures will remain at a fairly constant temperature. Back in the day, people dug root cellars and would "cold store" not only fermented vegetables, but carrots, beets, and other fresh vegetables as well. We have an old refrigerator that we leave on the "vacation" setting (approximately 40°F) and use it to store our ferments. If the ferments are stored above 40°F, they can spoil more easily. For many of my lacto-fermenting escapades, I cut whatever vegetables are hanging around into bite-sized pieces and mix them together with some herbs or spices, stuff them into a jar, and add enough brine to cover. See appendix B for recipes.

Our children are members of the first generation projected to have a shorter life expectancy than their parents.[8]

Pre-packaged food is processed, but not necessarily refined. Some frozen foods fall into this category. We home-freeze some fruits and vegetables, and sometimes we buy frozen vegetables. Let's face it: they are very convenient, although you do pay a price for convenience. Some nutrients are lost, depending upon the type of processing the vegetable received. If the vegetable is blanched, then any nutrients that are destroyed by heat would be destroyed, the same as cooking. Was salt added? That also may be part of the processing.

Neither of these things is inherently bad. However, some pre-packaged foods, like those offered by some of the registered trademark diets, are refined, processed, and/or chemically altered for preservation purposes and then packaged for your convenience.

Refined food is food that has been taken from its natural state and changed in order to use only part of the food. The easy illustration for this is grain. A whole wheat berry is a wheat "seed" that contains a balance of macro- and micronutrients. Whole-wheat flour is that "seed" ground. The more popular "white" or all-purpose flour has had the bran removed and lacks some of the nutrients that whole wheat flour has. And therein lies the problem with refined foods: they lack nutrients. If a person were to eat a diet of all refined foods, she would eventually suffer from both malnutrition and obesity, which illustrates the American food paradox.

When processed foods come under fire, the target is not mildly processed food, like frozen vegetables, but things like pasteurized processed cheese products. What is a pasteurized processed cheese product, anyway? A "trade secret." Once again, I haven't a clue, but there are many pasteurized processed cheese products out there, and if it is a cheese product, then it isn't cheese. They are so popular because they are inexpensive and melt into a smooth, gooey mass. They are a quintessential processed food. And they represent the tip of the processed iceberg. From breakfast cereal to cheez-ee poofs, we are inundated with factory-produced chemical confections that try to pass as food. Michael Pollan, author of *The Omnivore's Dilemma*, refers to them as "edible food-like substances." They have very little inherent nutritional value and yet compose approximately 80 percent of the standard American diet.

Look, any food that has to use "cheez" instead of "cheese" or "froot" instead of "fruit" should be suspect as far as its nutritional content is concerned. In addition to everything else, we need to be a nation of label readers, not commercial watchers. As an English teacher, I realize better than most that many people do not read carefully, that judgments are made by looking at the front of a package. Just because the packaging is in plain brown cardboard, with a kitschy image of a cow or an ear of corn, it doesn't mean the contents are natural or healthy. It is the job of packaging designers and advertising executives to make you want to pick up their product and buy it. That is capitalism and consumerism. It's akin to Calypso, who held Odysseus captive, and the lies she told to make herself look helpful. We are held captive by the images the media displays that we feel obligated to uphold. We fall for the lies sometimes because we don't know any better and sometimes because it is more convenient to believe that a food isn't *that* bad for us. Like Odysseus, we must show some fortitude. Stand up for yourself! Read the labels. Know the vocabulary. When in doubt, leave it on the shelf.

NOTES

[1] Robyn O'Brien, *The Unhealthy Truth: How Our Food Is Making Us Sick and What We Can Do about It* (New York: Broadway Books, 2009).

[2] Marla Cone, "New Study: Autism Linked to Environment," *Scientific American*, January 9, 2009, http://www.scientificamerican.com/article/autism-rise-driven-by-environment/ (accessed September 9, 2013).

[3] Annie Eicher, "A Glossary of Terms for Farmers and Gardeners," *Organic Agriculture: Michigan Conservation Districts*, July 10, 2010.

[4] Ibid.

[5] Linda Forrestal, "The Murky World of High-Fructose Corn Syrup," *Wise Traditions* 17, no. 2 (2003).

[6] Tom Philpott, "How GMOs Unleashed a Pesticide Gusher," *Mother Jones*, October 3, 2012, http://www.motherjones.com/tom-philpott/2012/10/how-gmos-ramped-us-pesticide-use.

[7] Miles McAvoy, "Genetically Modified Organisms," USDA Press Release, April 15, 2011, http://www.ams.usda.gov/AMSv1.0/getfile?dDocName=STELPRDC5090396.

[8] Zachary Bernstein, "Public Health Experts Warn Next Generation May Have Shorter Life Span as a Result of Obesity," *ThinkProgress*, May 4, 2012, http://thinkprogress.org/health/2012/05/04/478249/obesity-life-expectancy/ (accessed September 9, 2014).

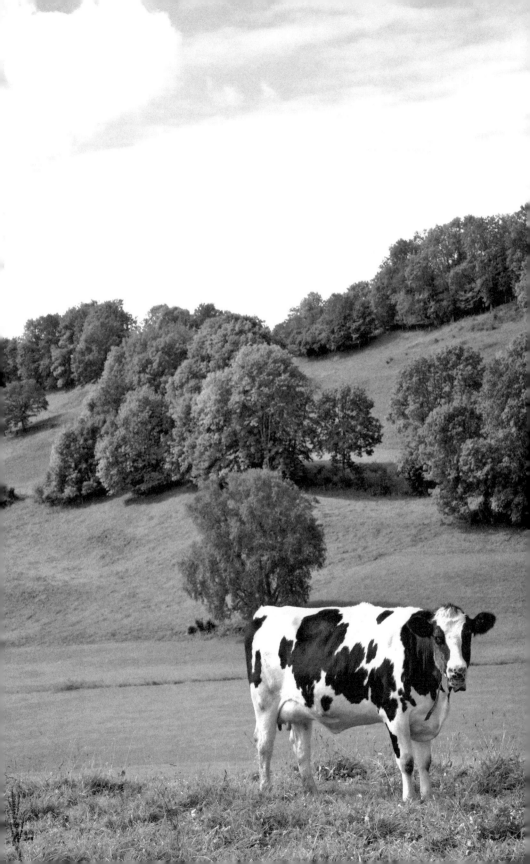

Reading the Compass

MAKING INFORMED CHOICES

5

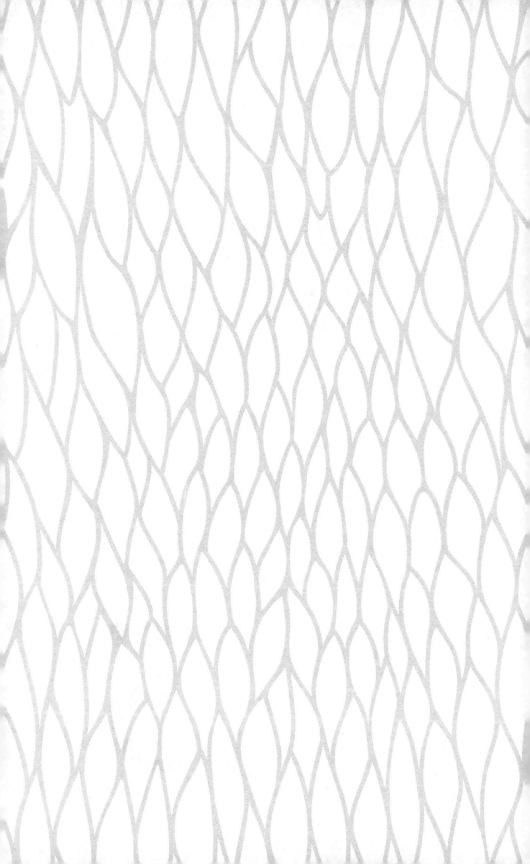

n science the phrase "a just-noticeable difference" refers to the exact moment an observer can tell the difference between two stages, when white becomes gray, or when a sound can actually be perceived as louder. I traveled through life doing the same-old, same-old, until one day I hit that just-noticeable difference, that point where I realized definitively that things had changed and felt compelled to say enough is enough. I think most of us are like this—you can tolerate someone giving you a bad time for a little while, but eventually you get to the point where it must stop.

The just-noticeable difference for my family and our impetus for change began with the birth of our daughter. She was a very healthy newborn, with fat pink cheeks and big blue-green eyes, and I was breastfeeding her. Things were going along fine, and then she got colicky. We tried the gas drops. They worked a little, but she was still colicky. We tried infant massage, we tried spacing out her feedings, we tried feedings that were closer together, but she was still colicky. The child seemed to cry, cry, and cry, and that was all. Sleep? Not much. Not for any of us.

At the time, my favorite breakfast was a grapefruit, peeled like an orange. Nothing was a better wake-up for me than the zesty aroma of grapefruit. One morning we were out of grapefruits, so I had oatmeal instead. And my daughter was less colicky. When I mentioned this to one of my friends, she told me that when she was nursing her son, he would spit up whenever she had eaten broccoli. I began experimenting. In the end, I had to avoid onions, garlic, broccoli, and cabbage; I gave up my precious grapefruits; and I sacrificed even my beloved chocolate for my daughter's comfort and an end to sleepless nights. (For the most part! Even now, over a decade later, she still wants to stay up "just a little longer.")

One mournful, chocolate-free night, after rocking my daughter for what felt like halfway down the Mississippi River, I rocked right across that just-noticeable difference: if what I eat passes through my milk to my daughter, wouldn't the same hold true for the cows from whence we get our milk? If what I ate had such an immediate and detrimental effect on our daughter, do the dairy products we consume have such an effect on us? And what if, because we had been consuming these tainted products for so long, all of this has built up in our systems so that we wouldn't notice enough to make a connection between the dairy and feeling poorly? I ran down the steps to share my revelation with Greg: He considered, we discussed, and I began researching.

What I discovered left me rather disconcerted: even the perimeter of the store can be polluted and deceptive. The perishables found around the perimeter of the grocery store in refrigerated or freezer cases are mass-produced. If I am looking at a cut of meat, and it looks nice and red, and the best-by date is over a week away, it should be fresh, right? But some meats are sold in modified atmosphere packaging to increase the amount of time the meat is red and looks fresh.[1] Farmed fish is displayed on a bed of ice to make it look just caught. Unsustainable and inhumane concentrated animal feeding operations supply our beef, pork, chickens (and therefore eggs), and dairy found around the perimeter of the store.

Produce

Much of the produce we consume comes to our local grocery from faraway places. For someone living in the Mid-Atlantic, the fact that the mango is not locally grown is a no-brainer. However, if it is

July, and the display bin is overflowing with big, red, ripe tomatoes, there is an assumption that the produce is fresh from the farm. In order for most produce to look perfect when it arrives at a retail destination, it cannot be picked ripe. Tomatoes are picked green, strawberries are picked green, peaches are picked green. If they weren't, by the time they traveled from farm to supplier, to the various distributors, to the specific store warehouses, to the individual store, the fruit would be bruised, battered, and unsellable. Those beautiful tomatoes in the produce department may have come from the opposite coast and been gassed with ethylene to make them ripe. The end result is a very beautiful looking peach, strawberry, or tomato that has a mealy consistency and very little flavor.

What about the display of locally grown peaches? Were they grown conventionally? If so, they may contain as many as fifty pesticides, some of which may exceed the limits set by the FDA.[2] While many of these chemicals are tested for toxicity individually, they are not tested in concert with each other. One chemical may be benign alone but dangerous when mixed with other substances. Chemicals hide in places consumers do not expect—even things labeled organic. Recently, the National Organics Standards Board came to the decision that the antibiotic streptomycin was to no longer be used as a pesticide application.[3] What consumer would think that the organic apple she used to make applesauce might be harboring a low dose of synthetic antibiotic?

Eggs

Conventionally produced eggs come from chickens that are de-beaked to prevent harm caused by stress-induced excessive pecking and set in cages to lay eggs. Each chicken is allotted about 67 square inches of cage space (by comparison, a standard sheet of paper measures 94 square inches).[4] The eggs are then cleaned by bleaching them in a chlorine solution and crated. They are sent to distributors to box, and then sent to the store. Do you want to know how old your eggs are? Look on the end of the box for a stamped three-digit number. This number is the Julian calendar, or day of the year that the eggs were put into that box. For example, today is 196, or in Gregorian terms, July 15. Eggs actually have a pretty long shelf-life—four to five weeks after the packing date. The carton may be labeled fresh and contain month-old eggs.

An eggshell is a semi-permeable membrane, which means molecules can pass through the shell. Battery-produced eggs are cleaned with chlorine. How much chlorine passes through to the egg inside? I used to get my eggs from a friend who lives down the road from me. I would take them unwashed and when I get home I brush them off since chickens secrete a protective coating on the eggs to keep them healthy. I now get eggs from my own chickens in my yard, a birthday gift that keeps giving. Eggs that are laid by chickens in clean coops with plenty of space are generally pretty clean, and a chicken that roams a pasture or woodland produces an egg with a deep golden-orangey-yellowy yolk. Yes, you can get commercial eggs with yolks of that color, as they have become prized by food enthusiasts as an indication of good flavor and better nutrition. However, some egg producers feed laying hens marigold petals to enhance the yolk color. This improves the look of the mass-produced perishable, making it more desirable than another brand of egg, but not its nutritional value or the living conditions of the laying hens.

Dairy

Commercially produced milk comes from a number of dairies whose main goal is to make money. The cows eat feed, which may contain genetically modified corn, soy, and sometimes chicken waste. They are given antibiotics. In order to increase milk production, many dairies inject the cows with recombinant bovine growth hormone (rBGH), a genetically engineered hormone. How much of this genetically modified material is passing through the milk? What effect will it have on me? On my growing and developing children? There were no longitudinal studies done to test the safety and long-term effects of this updated version of milk production. Remember, my epiphany was about my milk and my daughter's colic, which begs this question: what is a cow supposed to eat in order to be healthy, and therefore, keep the people drinking that milk healthy? Easy answer: Green plants, like grass. So despite that illustration of a cow in a pasture on the label of the milk carton, the cows who gave the milk in that carton may have never seen a pasture, or sunlight for that matter.

Meat

Most of the meat available at the grocery stores comes from concentrated animal feeding operations (CAFOs). An operation is considered a CAFO if it confines a certain number of animals (the exact number depends on the species, but it can be anywhere from a hundred to millions) to a lot with no vegetation for at least forty-five days of the year. The living conditions for these animals are not pleasant. If you have the stomach for it, you can check out innumerable videos available online from groups such as PETA (People for the Ethical Treatment of Animals).

I remember driving up I-25 in Colorado and being overwhelmed by an atrocious smell. When I asked my passenger what it could be, she laughed and replied, "Greeley." I didn't realize at the time that Greeley, Colorado, had a large number of feedlots, nor did I realize any of the impact those feedlots had on the animals or the environment. CAFOs produce an immense quantity of waste, from animal manure to carcasses, which can contaminate the soil, air, and drinking water. According to the Michigan chapter of the Sierra Club, "CAFO waste is usually not treated to reduce disease-causing pathogens, nor to remove chemicals, pharmaceuticals, heavy metals, or other pollutants. . . . Airborne particulate matter found near CAFOs can carry disease-causing bacteria, fungus, or other pathogens."[5] With so many animals being kept in close proximity, CAFO operators have to rely heavily on antibiotics to curb the spread of disease. Reports estimate that 70 percent of all antibiotics used in the United States each year are given to meat-producing animals. The animal wastes from these facilities are thus crawling with antibiotic-resistant bacteria. Evidence strongly suggests that eating meat produced in this way, or even living in the same community as a CAFO, can reduce the effectiveness of antibiotics to fight diseases in humans.[6]

The unnatural feeding practices for animals on these feedlots are also disturbing. On the average feedlot, the cows are fed waste: the leftovers from making tofu; corn kernels, cobs, and stalks; and in some cases ground chicken waste. The high-protein diet makes the steer gain weight faster, which means that the animal will be ready for slaughter sooner (and after looking at video of the feedlots, it may be a blessing that they don't have to suffer there any longer).

The Appeal of Veal

I realize what I'm about to say may be controversial, but please hear me out: we eat veal. We didn't eat veal before we began our food odyssey, but now we do. We, too, object to calves being raised in the dark, tethered down so they can't move, in quarters so close that most of the animals are sickly. Our veal was raised out in the pasture, consuming a combination of mother's milk and grass from the field. Our veal frolicked around in the sunshine and had a good life. Our veal had a much better life than most people's battery-produced chickens that had their beaks cut off, were raised in dark barns, and confined in wire cages that are stacked one on top of another so the chickens are pooping on each other. Among things that gall me is someone saying, with regard to veal, "Oh, but still! It was just a baby!" You know what? It was older than that commercially-produced chicken breast that only lived for eight to ten weeks in a tiny, cramped cage inside a windowless shed, and it lived a better life to boot.

One major grocer now employs a meat rating system, ranking meats (beef, veal, pork, and poultry) on a scale of 1 to 5+, with 1 being conventionally raised (in other words, animal feeding operations that may or may not be "concentrated") and 5+ being born and raised on the same farm in an animal-centered environment. I found that encouraging, until I looked from one end of the meat counter to the other, and didn't find anything rated higher than a 4, which is pasture-centered. The implication is that this is grass-fed meat, but "pasture-centered" means just that—centered on pasture, not restricted to pasture (meaning the animal could finish its life on corn, which adds fat and water for a heavier weight), and allows for animal modifications.

In one sense buying that steak rated a 4 is much better than buying meat that is rated a 1. However, where can you find meat with the highest rating, and be positive that the animal was treated with the utmost care? By dealing directly with the farmer that raised the animal, which is covered more in-depth in chapters 7 and 8.

Fish

At the fish counter, I see wild-caught salmon next to farm-raised salmon. Over-fishing is a common problem in many places, so maybe the farm-raised is better. But farm-raised salmon are confined to overcrowded pools, which leads to sickness among the fish and pollutes waterways with an excess of fish excrement. There are no easy answers as to whether it's healthier or more environmentally friendly to buy farm-raised or wild-caught fish, but the Monterey Bay Aquarium Seafood Watch website offers information about individual varieties of fish and makes recommendations based on their environmental impact.* If the supermarket were the only place to purchase food, I would probably become a vegetarian.

~~~~~~~

* Monterey Bay Aquarium Seafood Watch, http://www.seafoodwatch.org/.

In addition to the environment in which the animals are raised, we need to look at the refining process the foods around the perimeter may undergo. At the fish counter, that farm-raised salmon is usually "color-enhanced" with canthaxanthin, which changes the color from gray to pink. Mixed into the rows of fresh meat, you can find pot roasts ready to heat in the microwave. On the shelf just below the boneless, skinless chicken breast (a big seller, and usually placed just above eye level) are seasoned boneless, skinless chicken breasts (positioned at eye-level) that you just have to pop in the pan. In the dairy case, you can find individually wrapped cheese "slices" advertising that each slice has the same amount of calcium as a five-ounce glass of milk. That's great, since 1.5 ounces of real cheese also has the same amount of calcium as a 5-ounce glass of milk without the excess processing. But refining also occurs in ways we don't realize. I will use milk as my particular illustration for this.

While we don't think of commercial milk as refined, I believe milk goes through two separate refining processes: pasteurization and homogenization. I realize that most people would not consider these processes refining, but what then would they be called? The milk is taken from the cow, cooked and then pressure-treated. If refining flour reduces its nutritional value, is it any surprise that refining the milk does the same thing?

Pasteurization is the process of heating the milk to remove dangerous pathogens. I believe that pasteurization had its time and place in history. Prior to the advances that have been made in milking equipment (like refrigeration), pasteurization was an amazing advance. The process kills bacteria and sterilizes the milk. Along with the bad bacteria, the good bacteria are gone. The heat destroys many essential elements, like amino acids that make the proteins more available to the body. The vitamins that are destroyed by heating the milk include as much as half of the vitamin C and all of the B_{12}.[7] The mineral availability is also reduced. How is this for a paradox: we drink milk for the calcium to develop healthy teeth and bones, but the only milk that is readily available to the American public has been pasteurized, thus making the calcium less available for the body to use. Heat also destroys enzymes like lipase that help with the digestion and utilization of the nutrients in the milk.[8] What happens once the milk is sterilized? We fortify the milk by adding synthetic vitamins. The milk is stripped of its nutrients and then synthetic fortification is added. I see a pattern with our food, a pattern that is affecting every area of the American diet. We strip food of its innate nutrients then add synthetic nutrients to compensate.

Milk that comes out of a cow separates into layers: the lower, watery milk layer and the upper, butterfat-rich cream layer. That watery layer is "skim milk," which gets its name from people who, back in the days before homogenization, skimmed that cream layer off of the milk to use for coffee or on their oatmeal. Families who had their own cows wouldn't drink that skimmed milk; they would feed it to their pigs because they didn't think it fit for human consumption. And yet, many Americans today drink skim milk because they think it is healthier due to the rampant "fatophobia" driving our food system.

Most Americans don't know that milk naturally separates because most Americans drink homogenized milk. What is homogenization, exactly? Milk passes through a filter at very high pressure. The fat globules that form the cream layer are made smaller and evenly dispersed within the liquid milk. Well, that doesn't sound so bad. The problem is that in this state, the fat molecules become "capsules" for substances that bypass digestion. Proteins that would normally be digested in the stomach or gut are not broken down. Homogenized milk becomes a way of bypassing normal digestive processes and delivering steroid and protein hormones to the human body. Robert Cohen presents an excellent argument against homogenized milk in his article "Homogenized Milk: Rocket Fuel for Cancer":

In theory, proteins are easily broken down by digestive processes. In reality, homogenization insures their survival so that they enter the bloodstream and deliver their messages. Often, the body reacts to foreign proteins by producing histamines, then mucus. And since cow's milk proteins can resemble a human protein, they can become triggers for autoimmune diseases. Diabetes and multiple sclerosis are two such examples.[9]

Milk is an important food. And the dairy industry is just that: an industry. It is working to make a profit. Remember that box of mac-n-cheese with the long shelf life? Refined milk also has an increased shelf life. By refining milk, Big Dairy can consolidate milk production with fewer and larger farms and processing and bottling plants because the "time crunch" to get the product to market is lifted. As a matter of fact, you can buy milk in a box in the "area" of the grocery store (as opposed to the perimeter) because it has been UHT (ultra high temperature) pasteurized! Capitalism, at its best, works by getting rid of the competition, and that is exactly what is happening in the dairy industry today. More and more dairy farms in New Jersey are going under because the small farmer cannot compete with Big Dairy. Big Dairy wants me to drink refined milk, because that is what it is producing for economic gain at the industrial level. I do have a choice and I choose raw milk. I can't get it at the grocery store. As a matter of fact, I can't even get it in New Jersey because the sale of raw milk is illegal in New Jersey, which is a shame as it is something that could save the small dairy farmer. Luckily at the time I am writing this, legislation is in committee in New Jersey to legalize on farm sales of raw milk. For more about on-farm sales, see chapter 6.

As consumers we have become comfortable with anonymity. Even when we have knowledge, we choose in ways seem counter-intuitive. When Odysseus traveled to the Underworld, the blind prophet Tiresias warned him not to slaughter the cattle of the Sun god, a warning that Odysseus passed along to his men. The men however, did not listen. They feasted on the forbidden cattle and paid with their lives. We know that perishable food production is an industry. And just like all industries, the corporate structures within that industry are out to make a profit. When we are hungry we want to eat, not taking into consideration the consequences of the choices we make.

Oh, and a postscript on that rBGH milk: Because enough people were wary of rBGH and refused to buy milk from dairies that used it, many dairies have stopped using it. Don't ever doubt the power you have when you spend your money.

NOTES

1 Myra Armson, "Gas Mixtures Help Preserve the Quality of Packaged Meats," *Scientist Live*, April 1, 2013, http://www.scientistlive.com/content/23480 (accessed September 18, 2014).

2 Monica Eng, "Pesticides in Your Peaches: Tribune and USDA Studies Find Pesticides, Some in Excess of EPA Rules, in the Fragrant Fruit," *Chicago Tribune*, August 12, 2009, http://www.chicagotribune.com/lifestyles/health/chi-0812-peaches-pesticides_mainaug12-story.html#page=1 (accessed September 18, 2014).

3 Sacha Pfeiffer with Dan Charles, "U.S. Organic Board Bans Use of Antibiotic 'Streptomycin,'" *Here & Now*, NPR Boston, May 2, 2014.

4 Bruce Friedrich, "The Cruelest of All Factory Farm Products: Eggs from Caged Hens," *Huffington Post*, January 14, 2013, http://www.huffingtonpost.com/bruce-friedrich/eggs-from-caged-hens_b_2458525.html.

5 "Facts about CAFOs," Sierra Club Michigan Chapter, http://michigan.sierraclub.org/issues/greatlakes/articles/cafofacts.html (accessed September 18, 2014).

6 Marc Kaufman, "Worries Rise over Effect of Antibiotics in Animal Feed: Humans Seen Vulnerable to Drug-Resistant Germs," *Washington Post*, March 17, 2000, http://www.upc-online.org/000317wpost_animal_feed.html.

7 Walene James, *Immunization: The Reality Behind The Myth* (Westport, CT: Bergen & Garvey, 1995).

8 Ibid.

9 Robert Cohen, "Homogenized Milk: Rocket Fuel for Cancer," Health 101, http://health101.org/art_milk_cancer_fuel.htm.

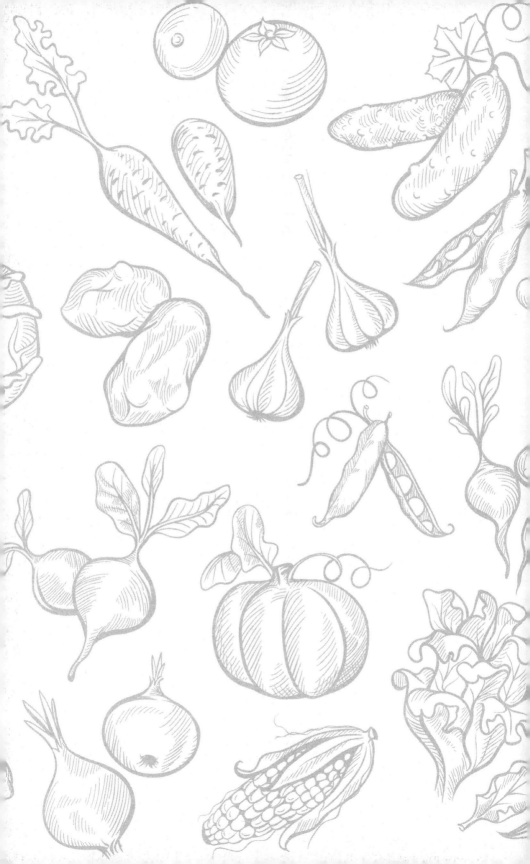

Part II

Embarking on the Journey

HOW TO MAKE A
CHANGE THAT LASTS

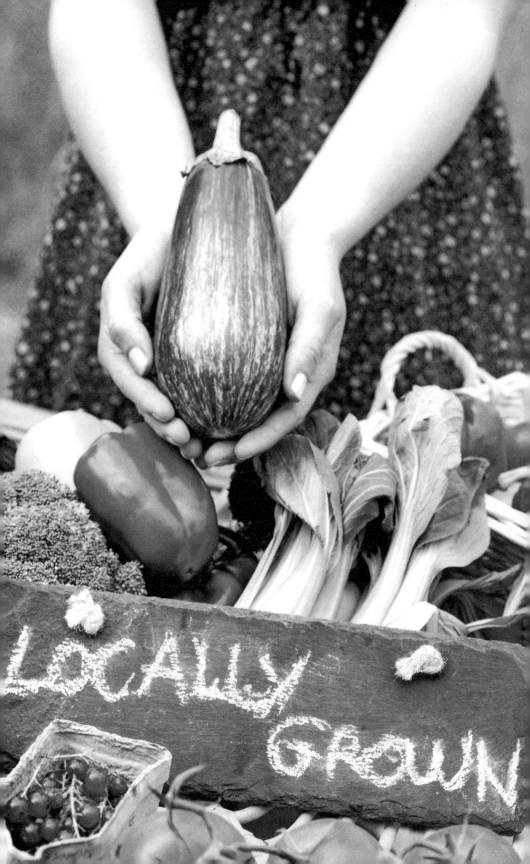

The Value of Farm-Fresh

LOOKING BEYOND THE WALLET

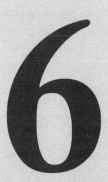

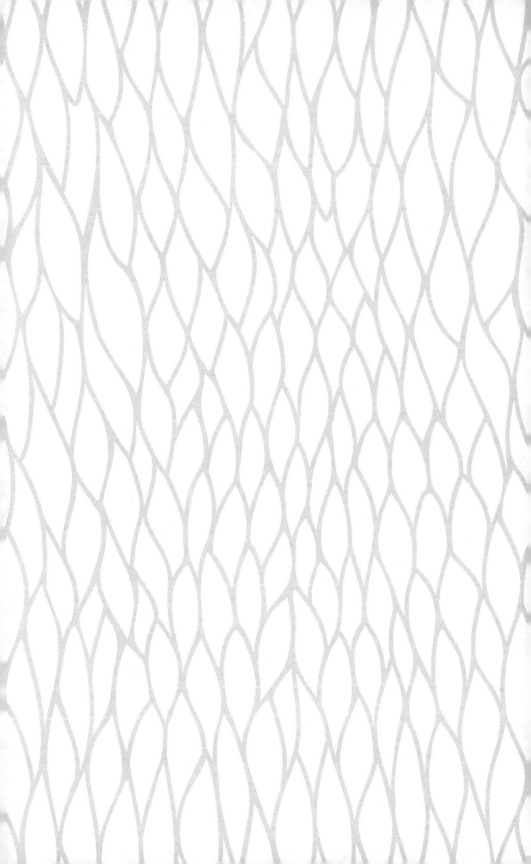

O nce I was married, I never ate commercial beef at home. My husband's family, who live in Minnesota, had been getting their beef from the same in-state farmer for fifty years. As insane as this sounds, we too began getting our beef from this same farmer, in Minnesota. Did I mention we live in New Jersey? My in-laws would pack it all up in their car and drive it out to New Jersey every year at Christmas time, and this was our supply for the year. We were all very sad when we were told that the farmer was retiring and none of the children were taking over the farm. We needed to find a new meat source, because the steaks we picked up at the grocery store just didn't have the same flavor or consistency, and we weren't happy with the rather expensive meat from a local butcher shop, either. It was all very depressing, but this cloud had a platinum lining!

Where does one go to find a new source for beef? The internet, of course. Even if you don't have internet at home, I would venture a guess that your local library does. My search for local, sustainable meat at last landed me at the website Eatwild.com, founded by *Eating on the Wild Side* author Jo Robinson, dedicated to providing research-based information about the benefits of choosing modern foods that are nutritionally similar to their wild, natural forebears. The site's directory of pasture-based farms and dairies led us to places like Nature's Sunlight in Newville, Pennsylvania, and our CSA at Fernbrook Farm in Chesterfield, New Jersey. That was back in 2004, and we found quite a few farms where we could purchase pastured meat products. When I accessed the site about a month ago, as I began the revisions on this chapter, I was awed by how it has grown. There are so many farms listed! How do you sift through? Slowly. Decide what you would like to try first, read through the listings for your area, and give the farm a call. The farmers are friendly people who want to do business with you. They will answer your questions. Just be aware that, unlike a grocery store, you can't call the farm on a Monday and expect to go pick up a side of beef on Tuesday. Many of these farms take orders well in advance (six months to a year in some cases) and raise animals to fill those orders. I will address some of the terminology you will encounter during your search in the next chapter.

The costs of buying farmer-direct may initially seem a bit daunting to the newcomer, but if you actually sit down and do the math you might be surprised. Our last pasture-raised beef cost $2.95 per pound and weighed 350 pounds—this was one side, or what farmers call "a half beef"—so we forked over $1,032.50. I know that sounds like a lot of money, but if you serve your family organic (which is not as high in nutritional value as pastured) ground beef once a week and use two pounds of ground beef at $3.99 per pound, you've spent $414.96 per year. If you serve steaks, organic rib-eyes, let's say, at $17.99 per pound, again figuring two pounds of meat, once a month, you've spent $431.76 per year. You have spent $846.72 on 128 pounds of beef. So, for another $185.78, I still have another 222 pounds of beef to use. That includes filet mignon, sirloin steaks, a variety of roasts, shanks cut for soup bones, short ribs (or what we used to call "flanken"), and more. Most farmers already have established relationships with a butcher, or they have the knowledge themselves and do on-farm slaughter and butchering. All of the farmers with whom we deal have the meat packaged into individual cuts and frozen when we come to pick it up.

You are looking at those beef prices and saying, "I don't spend that much on ground beef! The ground beef at my supermarket is on sale once a month for $1.09 a pound; I buy extra and put it in the freezer!" As I've said, there is a major nutritional gulf between conventional and pastured beef. More and more research is being conducted about the health benefits of consuming pastured meats. Grocery stores that carry pastured beef are charging upwards of $6.99 a pound for it ground.

When you purchase in quantity directly from a farmer, you will need some place to store your food. You must invest in a deep freezer. You can choose between uprights and chest styles. We have one of each. The chest freezer holds more, but it can be a little cumbersome to find what you want when the freezer is very full. The upright holds less, but it is much easier to see what we have on hand. I did the math with our first pastured hog: I calculated how much money we would have spent on pork at the grocery store (which would have been of poorer quality from a CAFO), subtracted the amount we paid for the pork at the farm and the amount we paid for the new freezer, and there was a positive balance. We paid a lot less for the pastured pork than we would have paid for conventional feedlot pork, and we got a freezer. In the past five years, our pork has gone up ten cents a pound and our beef fifty cents a pound, way below current inflation.

Keep in mind that ordering a half beef from the farmer usually means that you'll have a few months to set the money aside to pay for it. So budget it out. After you get the beef, your weekly grocery bill will go down because you are not buying meat at the store. If you put that money in the bank, the initial outlay (for the meat and a freezer) will be covered faster than you think.

Maybe you want to start with a share in a CSA. In a community supported agriculture system, participants pay for a "share" in the farm. If a farmer sells most of her produce at a farmer's market, there has been a good deal of financial outlay before any money comes in. With the CSA system, participants pay in advance and fund the farming expenditures (like buying seeds and paying for equipment repairs). Once the season opens, shareholders go to the farm or designated pickup location and get an allotment of food produced by the farm, or in some cases a few farms.

Just like different farmers have different practices, not all CSAs are run the same way. My CSA has quite a few crops that are U-pick, which keeps the cost of the share down. Some have tables set up for members to choose: two from table A, three from table B, or something like that. Others give you a box or a bag and that is that—no choices. You just need to ask questions and read carefully. I love opening day at the CSA because I miss my CSA friends, not just the farmers but the people I meet in the fields and the conversations we have over strawberries or green beans. We like being part of the community at the CSA—we see the same faces every week and have watched each other's children grow up. It is a place where my children can run and connect with the land.

Once again, there is an initial investment (our share cost $500 this year for approximately twenty-six weeks of produce), but our grocery bills went down by about $50 a week once the season opened. Financially speaking, this means we spend a little under $20 per week on produce for a savings of $30 a week. Over the course of the year, we save $780 a year on produce. As an illustration, our CSA grows amazing strawberries, of which we brought home about twelve quarts, including the "scavenging week," when the berries are about done. Organic strawberries at the grocery store were $4.99 a quart. That's almost $60 worth of strawberries! And no, we didn't eat them all immediately—a strawberry is very easy to freeze. Honestly, at $4.99 a quart, the grocery store berry would be too expensive for us to afford.

Buying local is a time commitment as well as a financial one. When dealing directly with farmers, a trip to the farm might take an hour or two or an entire day, depending on the drive and your relationship with the farmer. You should allow time for relationship building; making new friends is one of the major perks of dealing direct. However, the getting-to-know-you part can take some time. With one farmer that we see only once a year we expect to spend at least an hour or two just catching up, as friends will do when they haven't seen one another in a long time.

Packing up the car doesn't take too long. Generally the farmers are ready for your arrival and have the meat boxed. A half beef is usually six or seven boxes, so it doesn't really take very long to transfer from the farmer's freezer to your vehicle.

Even local farms tend to be farther away than the grocery store for most people, so transporting the meat safely is a common, though mostly unfounded, worry. Farmers usually will freeze the meat before you pick it up. We just cover the boxes with blankets to keep them out of the sun, and the meat stays frozen. Think about it this way: how long does it take for a two-and-a-half-pound roast to defrost? Now think about a thirty-pound box of frozen meat. I have yet to see a car ride long and hot enough to affect our meat.

Don't forget to allow time for putting everything away when you get home. Coming home from a farm and putting away a side of beef can take as long as an hour if we haven't cleaned out the freezer since the last beef. But don't fret; a half beef lasts us a full year, so this chore is something we only need to do once a year. While we make that time investment, it is time that isn't spent trying to inspect cuts of meat through cellophane packaging at the grocery store.

The first farm with which we dealt was Nature's Sunlight, run by Mark and Maryann Nolt. The Nolts and their farm forever changed our lives, and continue to change our lives every year. Before our first visit, we exchanged a number of phone calls, first to order the veal, then to discuss how we wanted the veal cut, and finally to get directions to the farm. The Nolts patiently answered all of our questions. The morning of our adventure, we packed a picnic lunch, snacks for the car, coloring books and crayons, the diaper bag, and the driving directions and set out for Newville, Pennsylvania. It was a sunny, warm May morning. The drive was three hours long. We turned down the lane to the farm and were greeted by the most idyllic scene: cows grazing in a pasture on the right and a team of horses running together in a pasture on the left. The barn and house looked like something that belonged on a postcard. It was so beautiful, it took my breath away.

The Nolts greeted us and invited us to take a walk and go see the cows, which we did. My children ran up to get a closer look at the beautiful cows. There was one curious calf that began to move toward us, but the wary momma got in his way. Then we got mooed at, and my startled son cried. It was kind of funny and we all laughed and then he laughed. And then the cow mooed again, and he cried again. And we laughed and then he laughed. Needless to say, we walked back toward the house before the cycle began again.

We had a relaxing picnic lunch, just admiring the beauty of the place and enjoying the positive energy. The Nolt family went about their chores, hanging out the wash, filling in holes in the drive with gravel. Our presence did not change their day. Greg and I felt a lack of complication, a straightforwardness about the farm, that made us want to begin to make our own lives less complicated. We looked around us and felt a reverence for tradition.

When we were ready, Mark helped Greg load the car with the veal, and I had a chance to speak with Maryann. She told me that they had started out farming conventionally. They slowly changed things over, bringing cows to the pasture instead of bringing the pasture to the cows, using less heavy equipment, and making the farm more profitable. They were just beginning work on a "milk shop." It was a very exciting time to visit their farm.

They had raw milk available, something I hadn't had since a friend with a cow fed me some, so we got a couple of gallons, some of their homemade cheese, and a dozen eggs. We piled in the car and drove home. The children fell asleep, as it was a little past naptime, and Greg and I had our first conversation about how complicated and busy the world has become. When we got home, my son was ready for milk, so I broke out the Nolt's milk, warmed it up a little, filled a bottle and watched my son guzzle it down faster than anything I'd ever seen him drink. The next morning, we had eggs for breakfast. When I cracked the eggs open, I was in awe of the color of the

Risk and Raw Milk

After our taste of raw (or unrefined) milk from the Nolts' farm, I was hooked and eager for more. I went on a quest to find a source of clean raw milk for my family. The Nolts are three hours away, too long a long commute to make for milk every week or two. I asked around when we joined our

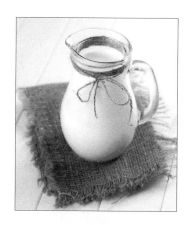

CSA, but people just clammed up. I got on the internet and searched for raw milk in New Jersey and found out why everyone reacted the way they did. Raw milk sales are illegal in New Jersey. Isn't this America, land of the free and home of the brave? Well, if I am brave enough to serve my family raw milk, why shouldn't I have the freedom to buy it? It isn't illegal to *have* raw milk in New Jersey, just to buy or sell it.

For a short while we had a steady source ("a friend of a friend who knew someone" kind of a thing). My kids loved it. We went through two gallons a week, easy. Then one of the links in the chain broke, and I was forced to go back to store-bought milk that was pasteurized, but not homogenized. It just didn't taste as good. We used about a gallon a week, and some of that was spent making yogurt.

Then a dear friend forwarded me an email about a farmer who had begun to set up "drop-points" in Pennsylvania to deliver, among other farm produce, grass-fed raw milk. I was so excited! I emailed my first order, drove thirty-five minutes over the bridge to Pennsylvania to pick up the milk, and met the farmer himself. We chatted for a few minutes in a heavy downpour while I transferred my order from his cooler to mine. I was very excited at dinner to pour my children each a glass of milk. They both looked at me, then the milk, and made that face, the one that says, "You really want me to drink that?"

In my best Mom-voice, I ordered, "Just drink it." And they did, and asked for more. Now milk is the beverage of choice at home. We drink a gallon every two days. It tastes good, it's refreshing, and best of all, we feel better.

I realize that many people will believe that I am taking an unnecessary risk with my choice of milk. However, more food-borne illnesses are associated with produce and chicken. Should I stop serving spinach? Most of the commercially produced foods that we consume contain a risk factor— the company producing it is more concerned with making a profit than a good product. Raw milk gets a lot of negative press because it is outside the mainstream. It promotes dealing directly with local farmers all across the country, which makes it an insidious threat to corporate food.

National chain stores and corporate brands issue recalls of conventionally farmed meat and produce all the time. In 2011 the U.S. FDA, Department of Agriculture, and Consumer Product Safety Commission counted 2,363 recalls, or about 6.5 recalls each day, for consumer products, pharmaceuticals, medical devices, and food. More than 13 million pounds of meat alone were recalled in 2013. Is anyone calling for the closure of market? Stopping the sale of ground meat? Food-borne illness is just one of the many consequences of our food being mass produced. This is the kind of thing that happens when four companies own 80 percent of the meat.

Therefore, another factor in our choice of raw milk is the ability to deal directly with the farmer. I know the farmer; I've seen the cows, the milking parlor, the handling of the product. If I get sick from milk, I know exactly where to go to confront the problem. My milk did not go through a distribution center that combines the milk from twenty different farms with herds of hundreds of cows. Conversely, the farmer knows that if I become ill, I am going to hold him responsible, therefore he does his best to put forward a safe product. This mutual accountability is what happens when neither the consumer nor the seller are faceless.

yolks—not the anemic yellow of commercial eggs, but a deep, almost red-orange gold color. I was excited to be eating truly fresh foods.

On subsequent visits to Nature's Sunlight, we delighted in a variety of cheeses, crème fraiche, yogurt, chickens, ducks, soap, and literature. We were introduced to the mouthwatering miracle that is spring butter. Not to be confused with butter that is made at any other time of year, the butter produced when the cows are feeding on the fast-growing grasses of spring is a bright, deep yellow and has a distinct flavor—the butter of butters. I would portion it out by tablespoonfuls on a cookie sheet and put it in the freezer. Once it was frozen I would transfer it to a plastic baggie, and then we would pull out a butter ball to flavor things that featured butter.

Our visits to Nature's Sunlight never fail to bring us new knowledge and leave us feeling rejuvenated. We admire the Nolts' work and greatly appreciate what they are doing for the health and welfare of our family and the environment.

One visit, I picked up a copy of *Wise Traditions*, the journal of the Weston A. Price Foundation, and a book called *Everything I Want to Do Is Illegal*, by Joel Salatin. These two publications changed many things for us. In Weston A. Price we found nutrition protocols that actually made sense to us (eat traditional, nutrient-dense foods), and in Joel Salatin we found a man who is producing the kind of food in which we believe and telling the story of how and why nutritionally dense food has become scarce. In addition, Mr. Salatin has publications available to help others follow his lead in food production. He wants to share not only his food but his knowledge as well, all in an age where people generally don't want to share their knowledge because knowledge is power—and most people are afraid to give up any form of power.

We see Nature's Sunlight as a pivotal place in our odyssey. It was the first farm with which we formed a relationship, and the Nolts made the forming of the relationship very easy. This farm represents the threshold we crossed into a better life. Our most recent visit allowed for quite a bit of time to talk with the Nolts as their son is now grown enough to be very involved with the running of the farm, and my children, who were little more than toddlers on our first visit, have become active participants in cheese choices and food loading.

Not all farmers have lots of time to chat every time you go for a pickup, but we have found that they generally want to be sure you are happy and have all of your questions answered. Some farmers we have met are all business, and conversations do not veer from the product exchange. Other relationships have become true friendships.

The farmers I have met are among the smartest people I know, and I know a lot of smart people. In addition to being book smart and highly literate, they are good at numbers and geometry, problem-solving and engineering, business and people, and, of course, producing food. They are lifelong learners who always engage me with discussions on the book they are reading or one they just finished. Why is it that the overarching stereotype of a farmer is of some filthy hick who wouldn't be able to find his way out of a haystack? Nothing could be further from the truth. Perhaps farmers being at the bottom of the commodity chain has perpetuated this erroneous and harmful stereotype. By dealing directly with farmers and bypassing the corporate commodity structure, we can raise society's recognition of farming to the level of professionalism it deserves. Where would we be without farms?

Herein lies your power as a consumer: you have choices, and all choices have consequences. When I evaluated what my family was eating, I had to view our food not just as a vehicle to deliver calories to my system, but as a piece of a larger puzzle. The industrial food system is a cyclops, with only one eye to see the world. If that eye is focused on profits, how can it see the dangerous consequences of money having become more important than public health? The industrial food system isn't looking into the future health of the nation. It is not looking at the consequences of the current system on the environment. It is not looking at the repercussions on our culture. A cyclops is arrogant because of its size, and sees itself as invincible. It will bully those it sees as inferior into submission through fear tactics. Lastly, a cyclops is cannibalistic and ultimately self-destructive. In bypassing the industrial food system and dealing directly with farmers, the money you spend on food goes directly to the person who grew it and not to feeding the greedy cyclops.

By dealing directly with farmers, I procure better food, bypass the industrial food system, and build relationships based upon mutual respect. Corporate food doesn't care about you; it only cares about your wallet and how often you open it. On the first day of school, every year, I talk about respect with my classes. I tell students that they shouldn't expect respect if they aren't willing to give it. Because of all the middlemen in the mainstream food system, we have lost a climate of mutual respect. For the farmer, the food products are trucked out to who-knows-where to be processed. The end recipient of the food is a faceless someone maybe thousands of miles away. For the consumer, food comes from a restaurant or a grocery store, and the person who produced it is anonymous. This does not foster respect. Consumers and farmers benefit from direct dealing because consumers know who produced the food and where to go should there be any problems, and farmers are getting a full market price for their goods, which they deserve. Both producer and consumer have a face, and this fosters respect.

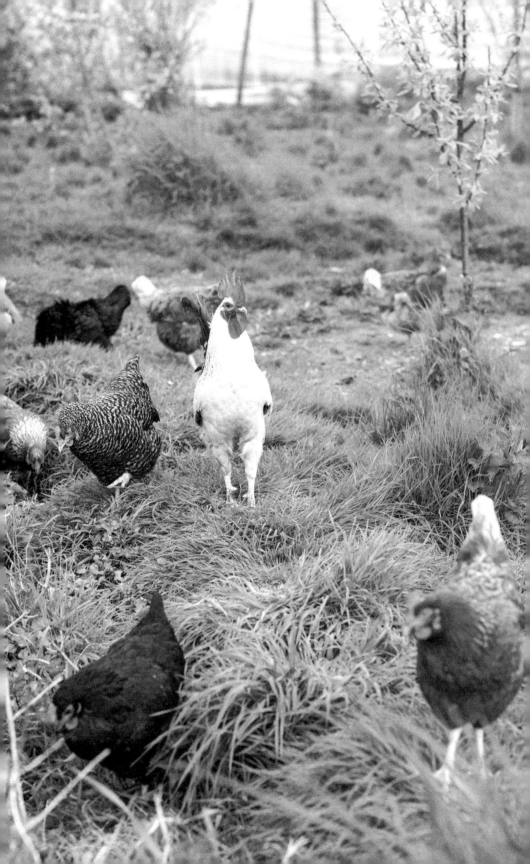

AGRI-CABULARY

THE LANGUAGE OF DEALING DIRECT

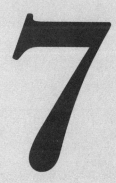

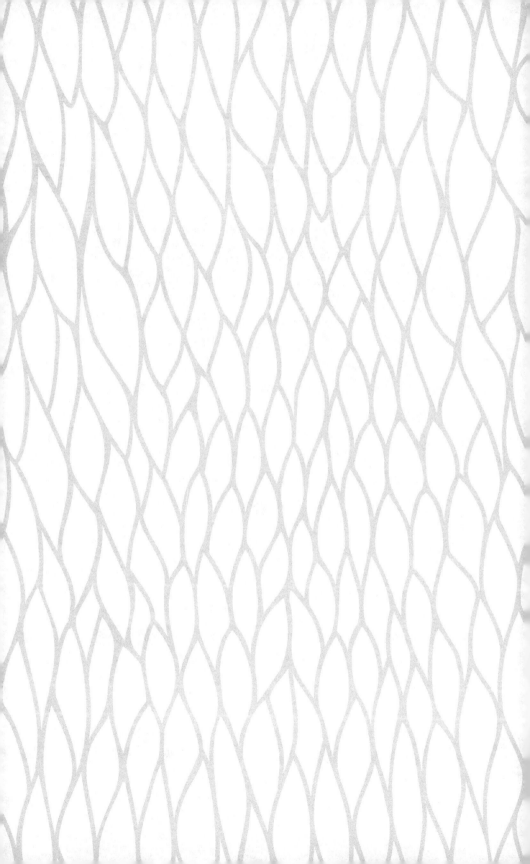

Taking into consideration the time and effort we put into our food, I don't suggest that you make a rash decision about changing your life in one day. Use a Thirty-Month Plan grid (see appendix A), do some of your own research, and make small changes, ones to which you can make a commitment. Part of what seems overwhelming when thinking about dealing directly with farmers is the fact that most of us have no knowledge of how a farm works. It can be intimidating to try and cross into an area where we don't even understand the lingo. Do you remember buying your first computer? Did you know the difference between RAM and ROM, or what a gigahertz was? I didn't, but I bought the computer anyway. Like most people my age, I learned because I wouldn't have lasted long being a low-tech Natalie in a high-tech world. So do some reading, conduct some research, but someday you're going to have to make the plunge if you want to make a change.

My search for beef led me many places where I gleaned a plethora of information about food and food production, but I was left with more questions than answers: what's the difference between organic and biodynamic? Grass-fed and grass-finished? Free-range and pastured? I found food sources, but in order to filter through the information, I had to become fluent in a new language. I thought I knew what organic meant, but there were implications far beyond my understanding of the term. On the other hand, just because a food is produced under organic circumstances does not mean that it's produced biodynamically or sustainably, or that organic animals have been treated humanely. The basics of the term "organic" have already been discussed in chapter 4, but let's explore some of these other concepts that may be less familiar.

Biodynamics is "a type of organic farming system developed by Austrian scientist and philosopher Rudolf Steiner in the early 1900s. Biodynamic farming takes into consideration both biological cycles and also 'dynamic'—metaphysical or spiritual—aspects of the farm, with the intention of achieving balance between physical and non-physical realms."[1] Biodynamic farming forbids synthetic pesticides and fertilizers and recommends dedicating at least 10 percent of acreage to biodiversity. Monocultures are forbidden, and no annual crops may be planted in the field more than two years in a row. In addition to its focus on sustainability, biodynamic agriculture incorporates a spiritual element into its farming methods, with a focus on ecological harmony and the celestial and terrestrial influences on biological organisms. Studies have shown biodynamic farms to have a higher concentration of beneficial organisms in the soil as well as more energy-efficient production than conventional farms, although their yield is lower.[2] A truly biodynamic item will be certified by Demeter USA, an organization named for the Greek goddess Demeter, who makes the plants grow every year and separates the chaff from the grain.

Sustainable agriculture is "an integrated system of plant and animal production practices having a site-specific application that will over the long-term: satisfy human food and fiber needs; enhance environmental quality and the natural resource base upon which the agriculture economy depends; make the most efficient use of non-renewable resources and on-farm resources and integrate, where appropriate, natural biological cycles and controls; sustain the economic viability of farm operations; and enhance the quality of life for farmers and society as a whole."[3] Buying organic is not necessarily supporting sustainable agriculture. If we buy organic corn chips, for example, we might be buying chips made from corn that was grown without the use of chemical fertilizer or pesticide, and if it is organic, it does not contain GMO corn. However, the corn still might be grown on a monoculture agri-industry farm, meaning that the only crop the farm ever grows is corn. Dealing directly with the farmer is the best way to learn whether food has been produced sustainably. When you are at the grocery store, one thing to look for is the "Food Alliance Certified" logo, which indicates that the food is sustainable.

Once upon a time in America, farms were family operations. If a farmer wanted to be successful, he had to know the best way to manage his land, extracting maximum profit for minimum expense. Sustainability was a necessity! If a farmer didn't want his family to starve, he needed to figure out how to make his farm sustainable. Yes, some farmers failed. But not all of them. Not even most of them—otherwise we wouldn't have any food to eat. We would be living *Soylent Green*!

How does sustainability translate into successful farming? First let's consider the land. The ancients knew that the fields needed to be changed up and allowed to rest. The concept of crop rotation is mentioned in Roman literature. The Hebrews used a form of crop rotation by giving fields a sabbatical year. Every seventh year, a field rested. A resting field was a growing field: the next year, it was full of grasses for the cows to graze. And the next year that field was ready to be planted, made fertile by some of the best fertilizer known to man (manure). Best of all, that fertilizer was free.

Rotation also refers to a system of interchanging crops so that what one plant uses, another puts back into the field. Back in the 1800s, George Washington Carver (of peanut fame) worked with farmers to replenish Southern farmland soil depleted by the ubiquitous cotton monocultures. Planting sweet potatoes, soybeans, and/or peanuts restored nitrogen to the soil, which both improved cotton yields and provided the farmers with additional crops that could be sold, used to feed farm animals, and prevent the soil from becoming depleted all at once.

Although crop rotation had been used all over the world for thousands of years, it began to fall out of favor in the United States during the so-called Green Revolution of the 1940–1960s. Around this time, farmers began to rely on chemical fertilizers to fortify tired soils depleted by monocultures. Industrial farming's overreliance on the chemical fertilizers and pesticides necessitated by these monocultures has trapped our agricultural system into a brutal and unsustainable cycle. In a sense, it reflects the increasing narrowness and specialization with which our culture approaches the world. For example, in medicine, the general practitioner has become a kind of triage that sends you on your way to a specialist for whatever your problem may be. In technology, one company takes care of the hardware and another takes care of the software. In farming, one farm produces one kind of food. This monoculture mentality helps us think about food only as an end product. Therefore, how it got to the table seems less important, whether it is a corn chip or a burger.

I've already discussed many of the issues with conventional beef cattle feedlots in chapter 5. The living conditions of CAFO cattle starkly contrast those of pastured animals, and these differences affect taste and nutritional value. Cows are herbivores, plain and simple. Allowing cows to eat grass rather than chicken manure is just common sense. The beef we used to get from the Minnesota farmer was grass-fed and corn-finished. This means that toward the end of their lives, the farmer would bring the steer in from the fields and fatten them up on corn for about a month before they went to slaughter. Grass-fed beef has been fed grass *most* of its life. If the steer was grass-finished, it was not fed corn at the end. If you are looking to be sure that no corn or soy were given to your meat, you need to eat fully pastured meat. Pastured animals spend their lives out in the pasture, the way animals were raised for centuries. What I find most compelling about this is that pastured beef is so much better for you than feedlot beef. Our modern production method for beef creates a food product that is detrimental to our health. One might assume that we have made advances that would produce healthier food, but the truth is that what is being produced is profits for the owners of the large meat processing companies and a lack of regard for the quality of the product. That seems to be a recurring theme, doesn't it?

However, pastured beef is very good for you, especially the fat. I can hear your incredulity now: "The fat!?" I know you've been told to avoid fat like the plague for the past twenty years. And I understand why—the wrong fats are really bad for you. Fats that come from feedlot-produced beef (the kind in the fast food burger, or the grocery store meat counter) are bad for you. But the fat in pastured beef has the same omega-3 to omega-6 fatty acid ratio as wild-caught salmon. Excessive amounts of omega-6 and low amounts of omega-3, as are found in today's Western diets, makes people vulnerable to many diseases, including cardiovascular disease, cancer, and inflammatory and autoimmune diseases. On the other hand, increased levels of omega-3, which would lower the ratio, helps the body suppress these kinds of diseases.[4] Pastured beef spends its life out on a pasture, eating grass, enjoying the sunshine. The meat has more texture, more flavor, and more nutrition than beef from a grocery store. Pastured beef comes from healthy steer; therefore, it is a better food.

Marketers want you to believe that "free-range" and "pastured" are synonyms. I love that term, free-range. The term itself conjures up an idea of a chicken running across a beautiful meadow, crowing, "Home, home on the range. . . ." However, the "range" for free-range chickens is in reality a fairly crowded barn, with access to three feet outside the barn. They are still fed corn. If they are pecking on the ground looking for bugs, they are eating their own feces, due to crowding. Free-range is certainly better than conventional production practices, but the point I am trying to make is that Jane Q. Public is given the idea that conditions are better than what they really are. Pastured chickens (or any other food animal, for that matter) run around in a field. A pastured chicken is provided a shelter, access to water, a nice green pasture in which to forage,

Using Odd Animal Parts

When you get your first half-beef, veal, or any animal direct from a farmer, you will have the option to get parts of the animal with which you may not know how to cook: the heart, liver, and feet for example. You have already paid for them, so it makes sense to take them and learn what to do with them. I am not a big fan of organ meats, not having grown up eating them. Greg made roasted heart for dinner one night and didn't tell me what it was, other than roasted meat. When I bit in, I was sure there was something wrong with the meat. My children, however, gobbled it right up. Since then we have tried many different things. These days, we have the heart ground into the ground beef—it's so dispersed that I can't taste it. Veal, lamb, and pork heart are not as strong and I don't mind them stewed. See appendix B for a few recipes you can use with these lesser-known meats.

and plenty of sunshine, an element absent from most commercial chicken production.

Because our beef and pork came from one farm and our veal and lamb from another, we were able to see that all farmers had different ideologies and practices. I found a woman who raised chickens for eggs and made a good friend in the process. A year later, we joined our CSA farm, Fernbrook, for produce. We have a regular source for fresh (raw) milk. We still purchase some fruits and vegetables at a local, conventional family farm, because we feel it is important to support the local farm. After all, life is about choices. I mean, which is the better choice, the local apple or the organic apple flown in from Washington State? It isn't an easy decision to make, but it is important for you to understand that choice and be empowered by your ability to make it.

When searching for a local farm, be sure to read the farmer's information carefully. Many farmers are not certified organic because organic certification is a lot of paperwork, but they use sustainable practices and eschew conventional farming. Often the only way to know is to ask. Once you have narrowed down your choices, contact the farmers. Not all farmers have email, and some may require a good old-fashioned phone call. Be upfront with the farmer—if you have no experience dealing direct, tell her (or him). Our experience is that farmers want your business and are happy to explain how their farms operate. And remember that the first call is not a commitment to anything. Just tell whoever answers the phone that you would like some information. It's always good to be informed.

Dealing directly with farmers is wonderful for many reasons, but for most people, I think, the idea of getting food directly from a farm is daunting. We are accustomed to shopping in a sanitized world, where food comes in packages. It's all very clean. The farms of our imagination, while pastoral and serene, are also dirty. But keep in mind that there is a difference between dirty and unsanitary. Farms may be dirty—nothing grows without soil—but a good farm will be sanitary in places where food is processed and handled. Most of these farms are very transparent in their practices and will let you see where the food is processed, and they understand that most people have never been on a killing floor, or have seen where their food is produced. We had no experience with this either. I wouldn't have been able to write this book without the patience of about a dozen different farmers, all of whom generously answered all of my questions.

On our first pick-up at the Nolt's, I was struck with this thought: Barns smell. Over the years I've learned that a pig barn smells different than a cow barn. And a dairy has a smell, as does a chicken coop. To an inexperienced suburbanite like me, not accustomed to the subtle nuances of farm odors, it all smelled the same: unappealing. Nowadays, while I wouldn't want to douse myself in "Eau de Cow Barn," I have come to appreciate, even enjoy, the particular smell of healthy animals. Outside of having a "Scratch-n-Sniff," I can't really help you learn to differentiate between a good-smelling barn and a bad-smelling barn. Trust your instincts, and judge for yourself.

To put all of this into practice seems overwhelming. Drive three hours to get meat? Drive to another state to get milk? Am I crazy? Well, maybe a little. But this goes back to what I mean by small steps.

We didn't go from shopping weekly for everything we need at the grocery store to dealing directly with farms overnight. Think about it this way: every small step helps. Each time you buy directly from a farmer, the money you spend goes directly into the farmer's pocket and you get really fresh food. When you buy food from the grocery store, the money pays for the store's maintenance and employees and advertising and insurance. The money pays for the distributor and transportation. And yes, some of that money goes to the farmer for his produce, but not much. The current estimate is that about 20 cents of every food dollar spent goes to the farmer. And the food in the store is not as fresh.

Small family farms are nearly a lost culture in America. The good news is with more and more people seeking out sustainably produced food, the small family farm just might make a comeback. My son told me that he wanted to be a farmer when he grows up. He was seven and I know he will change his mind about 17 million times between now and when he actually chooses what he wants to do with his life. But it made me sad to think that the conventional odds are against him. Luckily, we have good examples in our lives thanks to the Nolts, Farmer Jeff at our CSA, as well as the writings of people like Joel Salatin, who have all made a success of farming.

NOTES

[1] Annie Eicher, "A Glossary of Terms for Farmers and Gardeners," *Organic Agriculture: Michigan Conservation Districts*, July 10, 2010.

[2] Matjaž Turinek, Silva Grobelnik-Mlakar, Martina Bavec, and Franc Bavec, "Biodynamic Agriculture Research Progress and Priorities," *Renewable Agriculture and Food Systems* 24, no. 2 (June 2009): 146–54, http://journals.cambridge.org/action/displayAbstract?fromPage=online&aid=5636508.

[3] National Institute of Food and Agriculture, Agriculture and Food Research Initiative—Foundational Program, http://www.nifa.usda.gov/funding/afri/afri.html.

[4] A. P. Simpoulos, "The Importance of the Ratio of Omega-6/Omega-3 Essential Fatty Acids." *Biomedicine and Pharmacotherapy* 56, no. 8 (October 2002): 365–79, http://www.ncbi.nlm.nih.gov/pubmed/12442909.

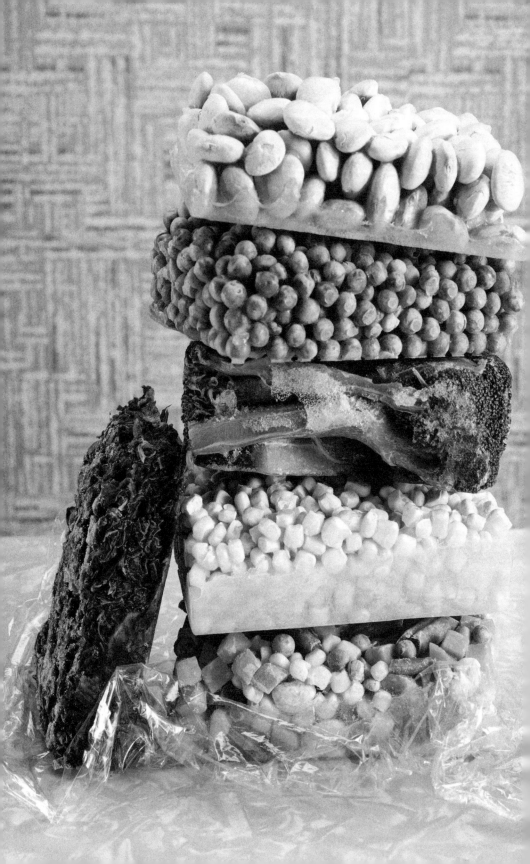

NAVIGATION

KEEPING SANE ON THE JOURNEY

8

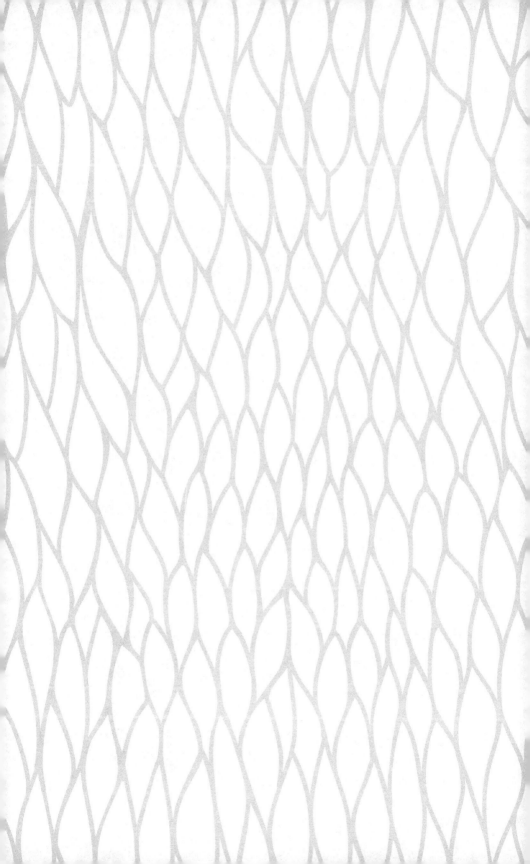

How does one make all of this work in the day-to-day? It's one thing to buy from farmers or a CSA and quite another to actually use the food and not just pitch it in the trash because it went bad. Logically, you think, "Well, I have the food; of course I'll use it." But the reality is that when you've had one of those crazy days, chances are you'll want to pop something in the microwave or call for delivery once you make it home. We all have those days.

When embarking on a new way of seeing the world, in this case the food world, sometimes avoiding falling back into our old ways can become difficult. As I have been stressing throughout these pages, making small, gradual changes and sticking to them is the best way to succeed. The next chapter of the book outlines how to prepare five meals in one afternoon. However, if you haven't really cooked a meal from scratch in the past ten years, or ever in your life, you may need to take this in smaller steps as well.

When you set up your Thirty-Month Plan, think about how you eat and how you can incorporate goals that will work in concert with your lifestyle. Of course, it's unrealistic to expect someone intimidated by her oven to begin making pasta from scratch. If prepared meals, take-out, or going to a restaurant is your dinner plan almost every night of the week, you may need to begin with preparing one or two meals a month at home.

More and more people these days feel challenged by the kitchen. The popularity of cooking shows has grown in inverse proportion to the number of people who actually cook. In a sense, cooking has become a spectator sport. My generation did not learn to cook at our mothers' elbows because our mothers were the first generation to enjoy prepackaged food. As time marched on, the industrial food system gained steam, and more and more of the cooking work was done for us. The last time I was in the grocery store, I noticed an amazing amount of partially cooked, semi-prepared meals available. In speaking with my colleagues at work, I also know that many people think that opening a can of this and a frozen package of that constitutes a homemade meal. One woman spoke proudly about the meal she fixed for her family: a frozen lasagna, frozen garlic bread, and a bagged salad topped with bottled dressing. While I applaud her getting her entire family to sit at the table for a meal, I was taken aback by the fact that in her mind the meal was homemade.

The world we live in today is so much faster than the world of our parents or grandparents. In my grandmother's lifetime, the world moved from horse-drawn carriages to putting a man on the moon. In my father's lifetime, computers went from something the size of my school (with not much function or capacity) to a cell phone that can tell me the weather in Zagreb, Croatia. If I need information, I can look it up on the Internet and have answers in a few seconds. If I want pictures of my children, I can take them and then print them within minutes. This carries over into food. If I am hungry, I want food immediately! That is a mind-set that must change, however slowly.

Changing how you shop for groceries will help the transition. Menu planning will help you generate a grocery list. I know many people already make shopping lists, but how many people actually stick to the list? How many "impulse items" do you purchase? Remember that the grocery store is set up in a way that makes you want to buy more items than you intended. It gets rearranged on a regular basis to keep you in the store longer, hunting for items and making more impulse purchases. When there is no food plan for the week, people are even more vulnerable to these supermarket techniques. Rather than shopping with a plan, we shop haphazardly and are left with odds and ends that may or may not be able to come together into a meal.

As a first step on your new path, try to plan out one homemade meal a week, maybe on a day when you have a little more time. Remember to keep it simple at first. Think of it this way: the kitchen is a new romance waiting to happen. Just like any relationship, it takes a while to get to know each other. It takes a while to understand the intricacies and patterns. There will be failures—I've had plenty of my own, from undercooked baked potatoes to overcooked dried-out chicken. Even following a recipe "to the letter" does not guarantee success because all ovens are different, and even stove burners on the same stove can vary in heat.

Another kitchen skill to acquire is stocking the pantry. Our pantry did not always look like it does now. Not even close. We started with one of those spice racks that were a staple of many American kitchens circa 1970, just ten or twelve jars on two little shelves. Now we have an entire cabinet full of spices and herbs almost as large as the cabinet in which we store our dishes. This didn't happen overnight; it happened over ten years. And buying one or two "stock items" a week won't overtax your grocery budget, especially if you are trading out pre-made foods. See page 133 for some staples of a well-stocked pantry.

I'm frequently asked, "Where do you shop in the winter?" The answer may surprise you: in grocery stores. Once the CSA season ends, we buy groceries like everyone else, just not the same groceries as everyone else. If you aren't planning on getting food directly from the farm immediately, then you will continue to get food where you always did. In terms of practicality, this makes sense. Small steps, right? Just plan for your trip to the grocery store to take a little longer the first few weeks, until you adjust to new products.

I cannot emphasize enough how important it is to read labels. Know what you are buying. Staying with the one-meal theme, you should try to purchase single ingredients for that one homemade meal for the week. For example, if you want to tackle a lasagna, then buy tomatoes, onions, and garlic, not pre-made spaghetti sauce. For a salad, walk past the bags of pre-cut, pre-made salads and buy a head of lettuce, some carrots, a cucumber, and a pepper. You get the point.

People pay thousands of dollars to have their kitchens refurbished, adding beautiful granite counters and stainless steel appliances, but for what purpose? To be a showplace? We have made the concept of cooking much more intimidating than it should be. In a sense we have made the kitchen into the six-headed Scylla, the fabled sea monster of *The Odyssey* who devoured sailors as they attempted to navigate her channel. The kitchen has become something to be feared and avoided. And who does that benefit? You don't need to slice onions like a professional chef to be a good cook. In our attempt to avoid the Scylla, inevitably, we run the risk of being sucked into our modern-day Charybdis, that whirlpool of easy food and the negative health impacts that accompany it. Like Circe, I'll warn those embarking on this journey to steer closer to Scylla. It's far better to lose a few hours a week of your time to cooking than entire years of your life to health problems caused by convenience foods.

You will have to start thinking about how you use your time and what you can trade to fit cooking into your schedule. How much TV do you watch? Give it up one afternoon. How much time do you spend on Facebook? Make your status, "Off to cook so we can avoid fast food this week." How much time do you spend at the gym? Give up one workout a week. Is any of this really more important than your health? Your family's health? I think that almost all of us can reconfigure our lives to find four hours to get healthier. But the gym is making me healthier, you think. The gym is helping you with a workout, but if the food you are putting in your body lacks nutrition, the workouts could be doing more harm than good.

I used to spend Sundays in front of the TV, watching football and grading papers. Once my daughter was born, I gave that up. Why would I waste a beautiful Sunday afternoon in October sitting inside when I could be pushing my astonishingly gorgeous daughter in her stroller? Why would I sit in front of the TV on a cold, rainy Sunday afternoon, when I could be snuggling and reading with my daughter? It was pretty easy to give up football. Easier than I thought it would be. What's more, I couldn't get over how much I could accomplish on a Sunday afternoon with no TV. I could grade more papers, I could work on the flower beds. I could play countless games of hide-and-go-seek with my children. Simplifying your life can actually open it up to joys and experiences you might have otherwise missed while sitting in front of a screen.

Now you know that you need a plan if you're going to make a lasting change for the better in your diet and lifestyle, but where do you begin? Even if you are not a planner this technique can work for you because the planning stage is pretty simple. In order to create a plan that will work, start by honestly assessing yourself:

1. Assess your lifestyle and your expectations. What do you eat the most of and why? Do you buy a lot of ready-made meals at the grocery store? Do you get a lot of take-out on the way home from work? Does your family eat in the car between soccer games and music lessons?

2. Figure out how you eat: mostly on-the-run, fast food, not-really-a-meal (for example, a candy bar and a soda), sit-down-to-the-table, or TV dinners on your lap. If you don't know how you eat, use the following journal template to figure it out. Write down what nights family members are home, who has what activity on which night, and what the carpool/transportation schedule is like. Make a schedule for each week and then plan menus to fit the week. Don't be rigid in the initial plan, but create a skeleton.

3. Take an inventory of what you keep in the pantry. Do you have a lot of mixes and pre-fab meals? Are there boxes or bags

in the pantry that you don't even remember purchasing? Do you have a variety of herbs and spices? Do you have cobwebs?

4. What is your eating style and why? Do you eat mainly chicken and fish because you believe that this is healthier than eating pork, beef, or lamb, or because you like chicken more? Do you eat boneless, skinless chicken breasts because you like it or because you are worried about fat? Do you skip bread because you have a wheat allergy, because you are trying to avoid refined flour, or because you are afraid of carbohydrates?

The easiest way to assess this is to fill in a chart, like the one shown below. Use the chart for two or three weeks. It will help you assess your needs. Once you have accumulated a few weeks of charts, look for patterns. Do you have take-out every Thursday? Is no one home for dinner on Monday? If everyone in your family has an activity that keeps them out of the house at dinner time on Monday, it is pointless to think that you will have a meal that everyone will sit down and eat. Maybe Monday would be a night for "dinner on the go." If every Thursday seems to lead to take-out, then maybe Thursday should be a "slow-cooker" night.

	M	T	W	Th	F	Sa	Su
We ate...							
We ate this because…							
Activities for me							
Activities for spouse							
Activities for child 1							
Activities for child 2							

Once you know how you eat, you can begin to create a plan. I am including some cooking ideas and sample menus in the following chapters, but they are meant as examples. It would be difficult to create five meal plans for other families because of vast differences in tastes, schedules, and food availability.

Remember to stay flexible with your meal plan. You may think that green beans would go very well with your pot roast, but sometimes when you get to the store the green beans look like last year's crop and the broccoli looks great. Make the switch! Or maybe you'll find something you've never seen before and want to try it. In order to minimize impulse buying, think about those choices. Be mindful of what goes into the cart.

We start the process by making a menu based on the CSA share (for the twenty-six weeks of CSA pick-ups) and what we still have in the freezer for meat. Here is a basic template:

Day	Meal		
1	Main Course:	Side:	Side:
2	Main Course:	Side:	Side:
3	Main Course:	Side:	Side:
4	Main Course:	Side:	Side:
5	Main Course:	Side:	Side:

We put this on the refrigerator and know what's possible for dinner. Notice that we don't list days of the week and weekends aren't included. After we have a meal, we cross it off. We usually compose this in pencil, because sometimes things don't go according to plan (for example the entire casserole lands on the floor or someone needs an emergency trip to the dentist). Weekends are up for grabs—sometimes we eat leftovers, plan special meals with friends, or even a special meal just for the family.

If your kitchen is uncluttered because it is empty, you may have some initial outlay expenses, but what you save by not getting take-out three times a week will surely cover these costs. Have you ever added up what you spend on restaurants and take-out in a month? On average, Americans spend $900 per person per year on take-out.[1] For a family of four, that would be $3,600 a year on take-out meals alone, more than we spent last year on all of our meat, purchased directly from farmers.

When I talk about a stocked pantry, I mean more than a cupboard with some cans of cream of mushroom soup and a few boxes of mac-n-cheese. I realize that it is hard to stock up when you have limited storage space, but when I began my journey, I was living in an apartment and had a kitchen that was about four feet wide by eight feet long with only a few cabinets and a fifteen-cubic-foot refrigerator with a little freezer. If I could figure it out, you can, too.

Back in my days of apartment-dwelling, I purchased vegetables from a local family-run farm. I would can some of these, pickle others, and freeze the rest. If I was making a stir-fry, I would cut up extra peppers and onions, toss them into a bag, and pop them into the freezer. Later I could take the bag out, defrost it, drain it, and pop the peppers and onions into whatever I was making. They weren't crispy, but they tasted fresh. This is what I mean by stocking. I certainly don't mean hoarding. No one needs to buy a hundred cans of tomatoes at a time! Understand the limits of your storage spaces and that foods have different spoilage rates. Most refrigerator freezers don't get cold enough to keep things for extended periods of time, and even canned foods have expiration dates. For example, we use up most of our canned goods in around a year, although I did find two jars of pickles last year that had gotten pushed to the back of the shelf. One was two years old and one was three. I opened them up because I was curious to see what the atrophy was like, and while they were edible, they didn't have the best texture. I'd still recommend using what you preserve within a year's time.

Keep in mind that not all store-bought canned foods are totally evil, and if the tomatoes at the grocery store look anemic, buy canned. They will actually taste better in your meal because they were picked and processed when they were ripe.

A well-stocked spice/herb cupboard does not have to cost you an arm and a leg. Many food co-ops and natural food stores have

Try This!

Still feeling nervous about diving into the sea of cooking? Try sautéed chicken: marinate sliced chicken breast in 1 cup of white wine, 1/2 teaspoon of salt and 1/8 teaspoon of pepper for about an hour (or put it in the refrigerator overnight). Slice two bell peppers and one medium onion. Drain the chicken, 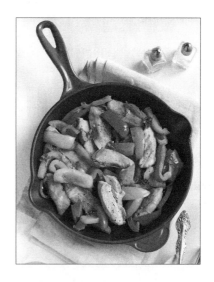 reserving the marinade in a bowl. Heat olive oil or butter in a large skillet over medium high heat. Press a clove of garlic into the pan and stir. Add the onions, and stir until they are coated with the oil. Add the chicken and try to get it in a single layer. Turn the chicken over when it gets a little color (brown). Add the marinade and turn up the heat. When most of the liquid has evaporated, add the peppers. Stir around until all of the liquid has evaporated. Salt and pepper to taste.

Now compare that to buying a bag of frozen add-your-own-chicken dinners. If you are deathly afraid of knives, then I can see why you would purchase one of those bags, but the truth is that it probably takes about ten more minutes to cut the vegetables yourself, and there haven't been any preservatives or chemicals added to the food to keep them firm through the freezing process. It is easy to do variations on this theme: add a tablespoon of dried herbs to the marinade, or 1/4 teaspoon of garlic powder and 1/4 teaspoon of onion powder.

bulk herbs and spices. In our area, we have many ethnic markets that have amazing selections of spices, and they are very reasonably priced. You can save a bundle by not purchasing these items in little glass bottles at the grocery store. But save any of those bottles you have on hand; they are great for storage. We get many of our spices through mail order. See the resources section for more information.

There are certain kitchen appliances, beyond the stove and oven, that will make it easier to execute planned meals. One is a decent slow-cooker. There are many styles available. I recommend one with a timer and a dishwasher-safe crock that actually fits in your dishwasher (a lesson learned the hard way). The other is a set of casserole dishes that will go from the freezer to the oven (which is what I recommend) or microwave (if you are really in a pinch, it's better than ordering take-out).

I also recommend a few other appliances and gadgets: a handheld blender (also called a wand or immersion blender), a food processor, a mini-prep processor (a tiny food processor), and a spare coffee grinder (for grinding spices). If you will have children working with you, especially small children, get an egg slicer, a rolling mincer, a small whisk (to fit the smaller hand), and a sturdy stepstool, so he or she can reach the counter. If your children are really small and working against you, wooden spoons and a sturdy pot turned upside down on the floor can help! But keep the children near you. Let them see what you are doing and how you are doing it. Even though it may be easier to plop children in front of the TV in order to keep them out of the way, one day they will be old enough to respect the process and want to help. Children absorb a lot of information when they are young—a lot more than we adults think they do. Making food preparation a fun, family-oriented activity will instill a positive association with not just food, but how it is made.

Navigating the kitchen is easier than you think. Just like everything else, you can master the skills if you start small. Remember when you learned how to ride a bike? My sister sat me on my two wheeler and pushed me from the back. I went whizzing down the little hill in our backyard and crashed into the house. I was petrified to get back on a two-wheeler until my otherwise not-very-patient father finally taught me a year later. Cooking is kind of like that. You won't master every skill immediately, but with practice and patience, it will come to you and eventually become second nature.

NOTES
[1] "Pizza Delivery Again?," *Daily Mail*, July 10, 2013, (accessed August 30, 2014), http://www.dailymail.co.uk/femail/article-2359696/Pizza-delivery-How-average -American-spends-900-year-food.html.

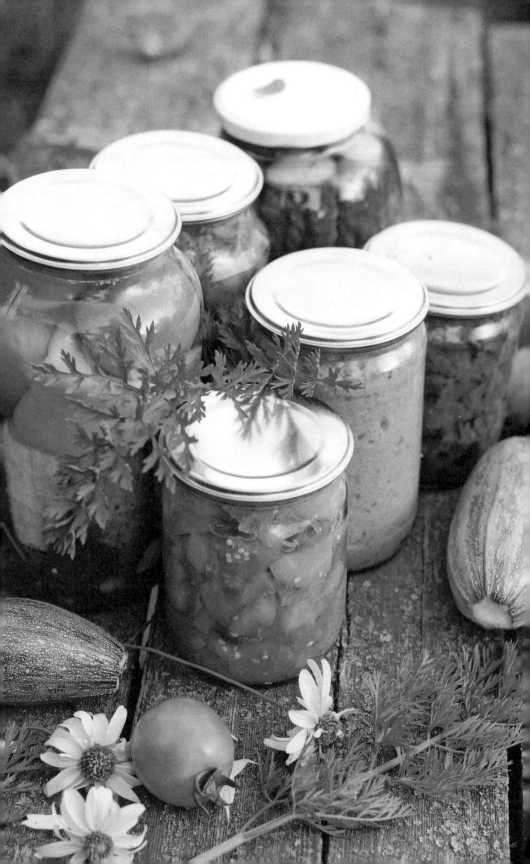

PERPETUATION

CREATING AND MAINTAINING GOOD HABITS

9

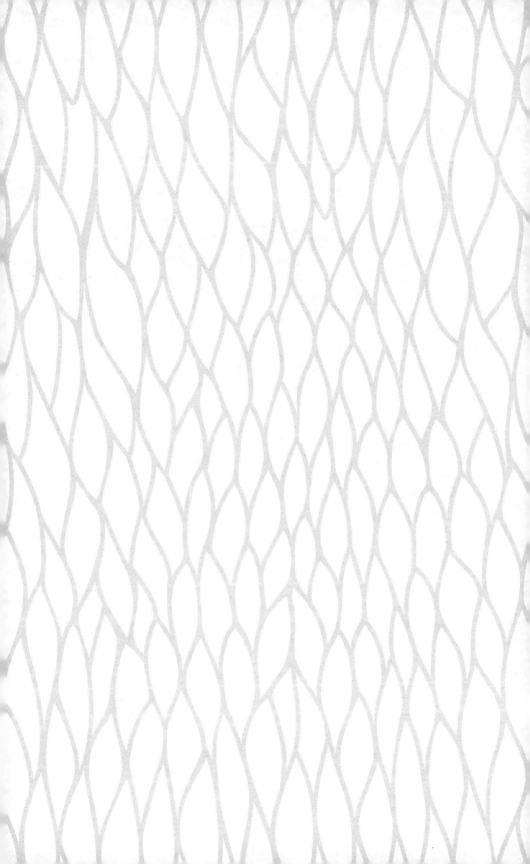

Working at my first high school teaching job, long before the birth of my daughter transformed my views on the relationship between food and health, my daily routine was to get up at 5:30 a.m., leave for school by 6:30 a.m., teach all day, coach every afternoon, and get home around 6:30 p.m. I was living alone and responsible only to myself. I knew I didn't want to return to the days of grad-school-ramen water retention, so popping open a can of ready-made soup when I got home was out of the question. While the weather was still warm, I was happy to throw together a salad, pour myself a glass of iced tea, and sit at my desk and grade papers or prepare materials for the next day's lessons. I was quite content with this routine until the weather turned cold.

In addition to my responsibilities as a teacher, I also served as a girls' field hockey coach at the school. We had a "no cuts, the more the merrier" policy and some years had upward of eighty girls on the squad. There were no indoor practices. Coaching field hockey from 2:30 to 5:30 in September is one thing, but being out there for three hours in October or November, especially on a rainy afternoon, is quite something else. When I got home, I wanted something hot! One Sunday, as I was grumping through the grocery store, doing my weekly shopping, I had a brainstorm: make dinner for the week. I'm not the kind of person who minds eating the same thing five nights in a row. I got the ingredients for chili, went home, and threw them in a pot. And every night that week, I took out some chili, heated it up, and had a nice hot meal. Stocking up on homemade meals became a weekly routine: cook on Sunday for Sunday night through Thursday, take-out Chinese on Fridays, and mooch off my sister for dinner on Saturdays (after which I would babysit her kids, so it wasn't total mooching).

I am an English teacher, before that an English major, and before that a book addict. I can't help myself, honestly. If I see a clearance shelf of books, I must peruse it. During one such indulgence, on the last day of my summer break, I saw a copy of *Stocking Up* (Rodale), a gem of a resource on home canning and preserving. I had never canned a thing in my life, so I am not sure what possessed me to buy it, but addiction is like that. I started reading it when I got home. The next morning, instead of paying attention in the opening day meeting at school, I slouched down in my seat and read *Stocking Up* (this was how I spent the better part of elementary school—reading a book rather than paying attention in class. Teachers are some of the worst students). By the time I got out to hockey practice, I was feeling like I wanted to try some hot-water-bath canning. I think the desire resulted simply from the challenge of trying something new—like the first time I ate sushi.

I had the good fortune of living near a decent-sized family-run farm. The following Saturday after hockey practice, I drove out to the farm and picked up a bushel of "bump and dent" plum tomatoes for $3.00. I took them home, washed them, cut them, cooked them, milled them, and cooked them some more. At the time, I was not a planner. While my first batch was cooking down, I went out and bought a few cases of canning jars and an enormous hot water bath canner. I had no experience and no equipment—I started cooking the tomatoes before I even had the jars.

I canned the first batch and got them in the water just as the second batch was ready to run through the food mill (a handy device that pushes cooked fruit or vegetables through a sieve-liked plate). I put up twelve or thirteen quarts of tomatoes that day, and I wasn't

Stocking Up on Stock

One major bonus of purchasing whole animals is getting the bones. Nothing can take the place of homemade stock, and nothing could be simpler. There are three basic types of stock I wish to discuss: brown stock (caramel in color, full-bodied, meaty flavor), white stock (light in color, milder flavor), and chicken stock. Once we began making our own stock, we started making a lot more soup. Rather than an all-day affair, soup became a go-to quick dinner: grab a jar of chicken stock, some shredded chicken from the freezer, cut up a carrot, and throw it all in a pot. When the chicken defrosts in the soup, add some noodles and cook until the noodles are done. Homemade chicken soup in less than thirty minutes. And dinner was made in one pot. Not too shabby!

Brown Stock

If the bones are not cracked, get out a hammer and crack them. Place them on a baking sheet in a single layer and put them in a 400°F oven for about 35–40 minutes, until they are browned. Put the browned bones in a stock pot, cover with cold water. Bring the pot up to a boil and immediately turn down to a simmer. Let the bones simmer for 24–36 hours. Turn off the heat and let the pot cool enough to handle. Strain the broth through a large sieve. Return the bones to the pot and cover with water again and repeat the process. You can get at least two cookings out of the same set of bones. Let the stock cool and scrape the fat from the top (see note on page 118). Processing directions follow all of the stock instructions.

White Stock

If the bones are not cracked, get out a hammer and crack them. Put the bones into a stock pot and cover with cold water. Bring the pot up to a boil and reduce the heat to a simmer. Skim the "scum" as it comes to the surface. This is just the blood cooking out of the marrow; it's harmless, but can affect the flavor. Scum formation will slow down after about 20 minutes or so. Let the stock simmer for 12–24 hours. Turn off the heat and let the pot cool enough to handle and strain. Return the bones to the pot and repeat the process. There will be very little "scum" on the second cooking. Processing directions follow all of the stock recipes.

Chicken Stock

We always get whole chickens. If we are using a chicken cut into parts, the back and neck go into a bag in the freezer. If we have roasted chicken, we save the carcass by breaking it into smaller pieces and putting it into a bag in the freezer. Eventually, we have enough bones saved up to warrant a pot of stock. If the pieces of chicken were frozen raw, I put them on a baking sheet and roast them in a 400°F oven until they are golden brown. If the bones are from a roasted carcass, I just put them in the pot. When all of the bones are in the pot, cover them with cold water and bring to a boil. Immediately lower the heat to a simmer and skim any scum that forms. Allow to simmer for 20–24 hours. Turn off the heat and let the pot cool enough to handle and strain. Return the bones to the pot and repeat the process. There will be very little "scum" on the second cooking.

To can: You *must* use a pressure canner for stock because it is a low pH food. Reheat the stock to boiling and ladle it into clean, sterile jars. Add the prepared lids and follow

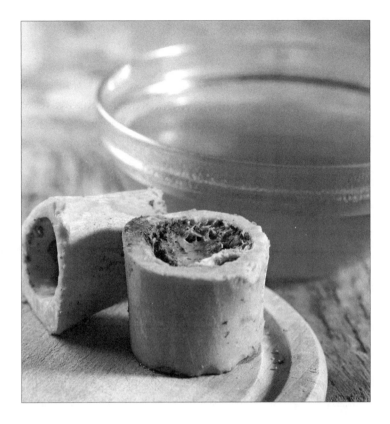

the directions for pressure canning meat (whether beef or chicken) for the size jars you are using and the altitude at which you live. Canners come with a booklet that includes a chart with this information.

To freeze: Ladle cooled stock into freezer containers. Label the containers with the type of stock and the date. We sometimes freeze stock in ice cube trays and then transfer the cubes into freezer bags. One cube equals two tablespoons, so if a recipe calls for a quarter cup of stock, we just take two cubes out of the bag rather than opening a pint jar of stock.

Note: We usually give the scraped fat to our chickens. We will save it for the winter and throw it out to them for a treat. If you want to make further use of the bones, you can dry them in a low oven until they are crumbly and pulverize them for use in the garden. Adding the bone meal to your soil pumps up the calcium and phosphorous levels and help with ailments like blossom-end rot in tomatoes.

sure it was going to be worth the exhaustion I was feeling. I had no energy left and still had papers to grade and lessons to plan. I flopped down on my bed and thought, "How did women take care of all of this kind of stuff and children and a house and cook three meals a day?"

Was it worth the effort? One bone-chilling, rainy November day, I decided that a pot of sauce and some meatballs were in order, so I popped open one of those jars of crushed tomatoes that I had canned that Saturday in September. Standing in my kitchen, bundled up in sweats, I was suddenly transported back to summer. I practically stuck my nose in the crushed tomatoes, I was so happy and warm! Yes, the effort was more than worth it.

The tomatoes lasted me into January. I became so accustomed to using those tomatoes that when I finally ran out and had to get canned tomatoes from the grocery store, I was in for a big letdown. They didn't smell like summer; they smelled like slightly metallic tomatoes. I knew that I would be canning more tomatoes in the coming year to last me through the winter, which served as my first lesson in seasonality.

Canning has become an almost meditative practice for me. I hadn't thought too much about what I do until I sat down to write this, as most of it has become second nature. Canning doesn't have to be a major investment. I went out and purchased a hot-water bath canner (at the time I was single and had expendable income), but you can use any large kettle as long as the jars will be covered with an inch of water while standing upright. Straight-sided pots are best so the jars won't tip. Just put a towel in the bottom of the pot (poke it down with a wooden spoon) to help prevent potential cracks in the jars. Some foods require pressure canning, so if you are thinking about using low-acid foods, such as ready-to-eat soups or green beans, you will need to invest in a pressure canner.

Always inspect your jars and be sure there are no cracks or chips, even in new jars. If there is a chip, there is a chance that the jar will not seal correctly, and there's no point in doing the work if the jars won't seal. No seal, no safety: the process of canning pasteurizes the food, and the seal keeps new bacteria from getting in. To ensure a good seal, do not try to recycle the lids—use new ones every time you can something. When I finish with a jar, I store it with a ring (screwband) on the rim. I don't know if it really protects the jar edge, but I feel like it does, and since the rings can be reused, they are already matched up when I take out the jars. When they start to get beat-up looking, toss them and get new ones.

One of the moments I love is the *pop* of the lids when they seal down. When you take the jars out of the canner, they are very hot. As the jars cool, the contents of the jar and the air in the head-space (the room you leave between the contents and the top of the jar) cool, causing it to contract (good ol' chemistry). The contraction of the contents pulls the lid down, creating the *pop*. Sometimes it takes a while. One time I made chicken noodle soup and processed about a dozen ready-to-eat jars. An hour after they were out of the canner, they hadn't popped. I was thinking that I was going to be spending the evening reheating the soup and re-processing it, but then, during dinner, we had firecrackers—*pop, pop, pop*. Every recipe has its own cooling rate, and the kitchen temperature will affect how long it takes for things to seal.

The summer after my success with the tomatoes, I expanded my repertoire. I bought a pressure canner and a dehydrator. I put up tomatoes again, plus peaches and applesauce, pickled peppers, carrots, dill pickles, corn, and my own ready-to-eat soup. The applesauce was great. The pickles were awful. As a matter of fact, I never made good pickles until my mother-in-law gave me her family recipe. It isn't in the book; it's a family secret. We must respect family secrets.

I learned to love the dehydrator. Dehydrating itself is one of the easiest preservation methods. I know people who have built solar dehydrators, dehydrate on baskets in the backyard, or use an oven turned to a very low temperature for dehydrating. However, getting a food dehydrator, an appliance made specifically for this purpose, makes the process easier. The variety, quality, and price of this appliance can vary from under $100 to over $1,000. I purchased a dehydrator at a thrift store for $15 about twenty years ago and it is still functioning perfectly.

In the beginning, I dried mostly fruit: apple rings and peach slices. When I had access to fresh herbs, I started drying them, too. Nothing could be easier, and it gave us fresh supplies each year. At the end of summer, I cut all of the remaining leaves from the herb plants and put them on the dehydrator. Cherry tomatoes are excellent—I have the kids poke them with a toothpick and dry them. They can be used in salads as is or rehydrated and used in any recipe that calls for dried tomatoes.

The most important advice for dehydrating food is to use the freshest foods you can. Wash everything thoroughly to be sure it is clean and remove any blemishes. When you cut or slice the food, make the pieces as even as you can so everything dries at the same rate. Larger pieces will take longer to dry. If you are put off by the brownish color caused by oxidation, you can dip things like apples in a solution of 1 tablespoon of lemon juice and 1 cup of water before placing them on the dehydrator tray. Do not crowd the food; make sure that there is enough space for air to circulate around the pieces. One way to involve small children is to dry strawberries. A child can slice the fruit using an egg slicer. A ripe strawberry is as soft as a boiled egg (just be sure to remove the green stem). And my children had fun arranging the slices on the dehydrator trays.

My initial interest in preserving food taught me about food having seasons. I thought summer equals tomatoes. So every time I went to the farm, I was looking for tomatoes. This started in June. I had no idea that Jersey field tomatoes weren't in abundance until mid-August. But when I went to the farm in June I found other things, like blueberries to be made into pancake syrup and dried for snacks, and in July there were peppers to be pickled (both hot and sweet). After a morning of canning I would invite my neighbor in to see my jars all lined up on the table cooling. She would laugh at me and call me crazy. However, in the winter of the mega ice storms, she was happy to share in a pot of soup out of my cupboard.

While I began to preserve a lot of my own food, I don't want you to think that I was super healthy—I certainly ate my share of junk food. Like I said, I had a weekly Chinese take-out habit, loved cheesesteaks (still do), and have a deep love for the Tastykake Butterscotch Krimpet (only the best snack cake ever). But most of my meals were homemade. I bought a majority of my food from local farms in season. I felt good about my food and I continued to can, freeze, and dehydrate. I had great successes, like the sugar-free applesauce, as well as abject failures, like the peach leather that went from goopy to hard as a rock in no time flat.

Even with the failures, I enjoyed the sense of accomplishment each time I mastered a new technique. Keep in mind that I didn't start this all by changing my whole life. I started by canning one thing: tomatoes. When I began canning my ready-to-eat soup, it took only about an extra hour, and I saved a lot of money. Rather than making one pot of soup, I made two. One went into jars and got processed and the other I ate that week. My whole pot of soup probably cost me $3 or $4. So rather than $1 for a pint of soup from the store that I would have to reconstitute, I paid $.30 for homemade. Bonus: it tasted great—not like metal mush.

Does this all seem a little overwhelming? I hope not. My advice is not to start with an entire bushel of tomatoes. If you just want to experiment, try canning only a dozen or so plum tomatoes. Another good starting place is jam. When fruit is in season and inexpensive, it makes sense to cook down some preserves. There are recipes in appendix B, and other resources are listed in the back of the book. The nice thing about jam is that you can "small batch" and not have an entire day devoted to canning. Last summer I made jam every morning for about a week. I began around 7, cooked breakfast for everyone, and was cleaned up by 9:30, just as everyone was finishing morning chores. Each batch yielded about eight to ten half-pint jars, and we had six or seven varieties of jam to eat all fall and winter, plus extras for holiday gifts.

You could also begin by just considering what you use on a regular basis. What is one item that you could make at home? Do you eat granola on top of yogurt? Granola is easy to make. How about pesto? If you ever grew basil, you know that at some point it just goes crazy. Strip off all of the leaves, pack them into the bowl of the food processor along with six to seven cloves of garlic (chopped), and about half a cup of pine nuts. Pulse the food processor to get things started and then drizzle in about half a cup of olive oil. When the mixture is pasty, stop processing, and add salt and pepper to taste. Scrape it out of the processor and into some ice-cube trays. It will take about a day to freeze through. Then you can pop the cubes out of the trays and store them in a freezer bag in the freezer. One cube equals two tablespoons. For pasta with pesto, take out four pesto cubes. Cook the pasta, strain it, and put it back in the hot pot. Add the thawed pesto cubes and mix it thoroughly. Talk about a fast, easy dinner.

Once you begin to preserve your own food, keep a list of what you have on hand. Ours is taped to the inside door of the cupboard. One of the saddest things that can happen is finding a bag of buggy dried tomatoes in the cupboard from three years ago because you forgot you had them! Sometimes when we are lacking inspiration for the weekly menu, we open up the cupboard to look at the list of what we have on hand and let those ingredients drive the menu.

Where should you begin? Only you can answer that question, and once you complete a Thirty-Month Plan, you will probably have an answer. Anxious to get started? Try this: the next time you go to the grocery store, buy two or three vanilla beans, and a half liter of cheap vodka. When you get home, slice the vanilla beans, put them in a jar, and cover them with the vodka. Put the lid on the jar and put it in a cupboard for about a month. Every once in a while, give the jar a shake. After a month, your homemade vanilla extract will be ready to use. You say, "Wait a minute, Natalie! You said 'anxious to get started' which implies an immediate result." Yeah, well that's part of the point: start small, take it slow, and be patient.

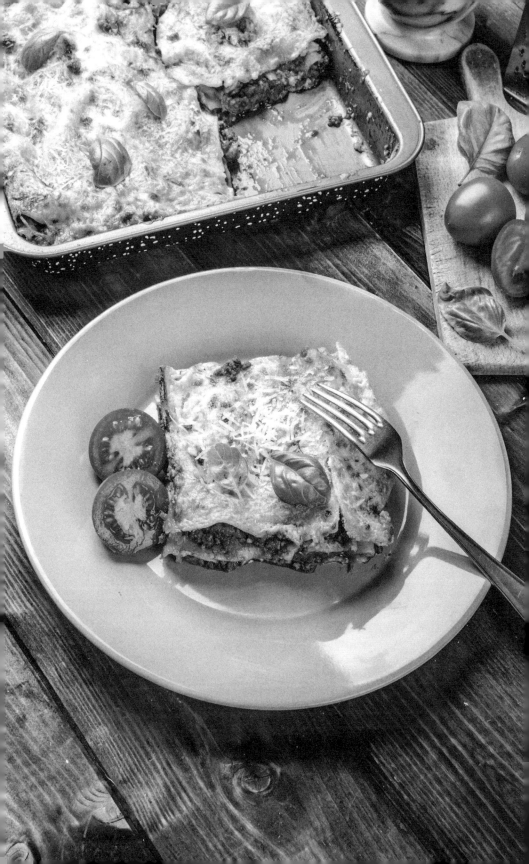

Taking the First Step

TURNING THEORY INTO PRACTICE

10

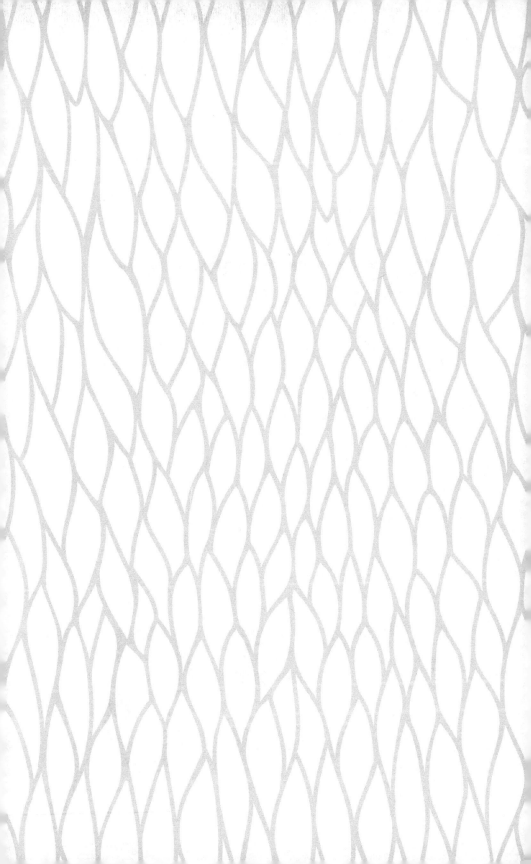

Right now you're probably thinking, "Okay, Natalie, this all looks great on paper, but so does Communism. How can we make this work in the real world?" When I was taking my undergraduate Introduction to Education class, I had already worked as a substitute teacher for a year and completed half of my education classes (I have a tendency not to complete things in the prescribed order). I would shudder every time some uninitiated future teacher would volunteer what her classroom would be like, full of unicorns and sunbeams. And I would shake my head and wonder, "What are you going to do the first time someone vomits on you? And when a fistfight breaks out, what will you do then?" The expectations of these naive aspiring teachers were worlds away from the realities of the classroom, but the only way to really get a feel for teaching is by doing. Once they set foot in the classroom, it was sink or swim. You, too may feel worlds away from sustainably produced home-cooked meals right now, but the only way to find out if you can do it is by trying it out yourself and keeping at it.

We keep our home-cooked habit going by cooking for the week on Sunday or making doubles and freezing them for future use. Making lasagna is a task, but it only takes about five more minutes total to make two rather than one, so I make two and put one in the freezer. The same goes for things like chili, soup, and spaghetti sauce. And here's a great hint for chili and soup: get containers that fit inside your slow cooker, and freeze the food in those. On nights when you want to serve them for dinner, take the container out of the freezer, run it under some water, and pop the frozen block into a cold slow cooker. Set it to cook for eight hours on low. It will defrost and then slowly cook and be ready when you get home.

Therefore on Sunday afternoon, we get our act together for the week. We put laundry away (well, sometimes; some weeks, we just pull things out of the piles that are still on the dining room table), we clean out papers from our bookbags, we change the sheets on the beds and straighten up our rooms, I bake bread for lunches for the week, and we get a head start on our dinners for the week.

We always consult the calendar first. Are there any special events in the coming week? Is it the week of the winter musical program? The second grade dinosaur show? The book fair? Then we consider the normal schedule: Cub Scout pack meeting means an early dinner; Hebrew school a late dinner; and Cub Scout pack meeting *and* Hebrew school means half of the family eating earlier and the other half eating later. In the summer, since we live without air conditioning, we also consult the weather forecast. If it's going to be hot, we don't want to be standing over a hot stove or turning on the oven.

Next we decide how many dinners can be made on the night we plan to eat them and how many should be prepared early to avoid the lure of being lazy and getting take-out. For my sample five meals, I am going to use a very busy week, one in which no meals could be fully prepared the night we are going to eat them. One night the plan is for a meal where half of the family eats at one time and the other at another time. One night is a dinner-on-the-go.

Here is the menu for my sample week:

Day	Meal		
1	Main: buffalo chicken wraps	Side:	Side:
2	Main: Lebanese-style lentil soup	Side: sliced raw veggies with yogurt	Side: pickled greens
3	Main: pot roast	Side: rice	Side: sauerkraut
4	Main: meatloaf	Side: kasha	Side: broccoli
5	Main: baked monkfish	Side: baked potato	Side: corn relish

Begin by assembling all of the ingredients you will need for each meal on the counter or kitchen table. Get out all of the kitchen equipment you will need, like a food processor, hand blender, mixing bowls, etc. For my sample week, I will need the following:

1 chicken	1 chuck roast	baking powder
beef stock	bread for bread crumbs	broccoli
butter	chicken stock	chicken stock
crushed tomatoes	eggs	garlic
ground meat	kasha	lavash bread or pita
lemons	lettuce	monkfish
nutmeg	olive oil	onions
pepper	plain yogurt	potatoes
raw vegetables	red lentils	red wine
salt	soy sauce	Tabasco sauce
tomatoes	water	whole allspice berries

I look at the meals I am making and determine the order in which to proceed. I want to make the most out of my food processor and not have to stop to wash it in between, so I want to go from dry processing (bread crumbs for the meatloaf) to wet (everything else). Then I look at things in terms of time and types of preparation. Most weeks, this entire process, from assembling ingredients to cleaning up, takes anywhere from two to four hours, depending on what I am making and who is helping. When all four of us are in the kitchen, it goes very quickly.

- Turn the oven on to 200°F. Break up the bread and place it on a cookie sheet and put it in the oven to dry.
- Put 2 cups of lentils in water to soak.
- If you are using a whole chicken, cut up the chicken. Place the back, neck, and wing tips in a freezer bag to use to make stock another week. Put them in the freezer.
- Rub the chicken with butter or olive oil and then season with salt and pepper.
- Take the bread out of the oven and turn the oven up to 350°F. Put the bread in the bowl of the food processor.
- Put the chicken on the cookie sheet and place it in the oven. Set the timer for 45 minutes.
- Scrub the potatoes and put them in the oven.
- The bread should be cool by now, so process the bread to crumbs. Put them in a bowl.
- Process about 4 medium onions. Put them in a bowl and cover the bowl with a plate to keep you from crying.
- Chop 4 cloves of garlic.
- Place a 6-quart pot on the stove. Heat up about 2–3 tablespoons of olive oil. Put in about half the processed onions and two cloves of garlic. Slowly sauté the onions and garlic. Add the juice of one lemon and 7–8 whole allspice berries.
- Drain the lentils and add them to the pot. Stir until everything looks nice and shiny, and then add 2 quarts of chicken stock. Stir, lower the heat, and put a lid on it. While you are working

on the other meals, check in on the soup every so often and give a stir. Eventually the red lentils will begin to burst.

- Put half of the ground meat and half of the bread crumbs in the food processor. Add a little chopped garlic, half of what is left of the onions, one egg, and a teaspoon of baking powder. Process until the ingredients are thoroughly mixed. Empty this into a bowl and repeat the process with the remaining meat, onions, and garlic, a teaspoon of baking powder, and one egg. Combine the two mixtures and press into a greased loaf pan. Place this in the oven.

- When the timer goes off, remove the potatoes. If the chicken is done, take it out of the oven and let it cool. If it isn't (which it should be), check it every five minutes. Let the potatoes cool.

- Grease the bottom of the crock of the slow cooker. Place about a cup of sliced onions in the bottom. Place a chuck roast (or any other roast that will stand up to braising) on top of the onions. Pour in a can of crushed tomatoes, a cup of beef stock, one tablespoon of soy sauce, and about half a cup of red wine. Put another cup of sliced onions on top of the roast. Put the lid on the crock and put the whole deal into the freezer.

- In a heavy skillet, toast one cup of kasha. It will smell very nutty. Transfer it to another bowl (like the one that held the bread crumbs earlier). While the kasha cools, put 2 cups of liquid in a pot to heat up—one of my grandmothers used water, the other chicken stock. Beat an egg, and when the kasha is cooled, mix it in the egg. Reheat the skillet and cook the egg and kasha, stirring constantly, so the egg cooks and the kasha kernels are separated. Put this into the boiling liquid and stir gently until it comes back to a boil. Lower the heat, cover, and let it simmer for about 30 minutes.

- While the kasha is simmering, check the meatloaf. If it is pulling away from the sides of the pan, remove it from the oven. If not, check on it every 10 minutes or so. Take it out of the oven and let it cool.

- The potatoes have probably cooled by now, so wrap them in foil and put them in the freezer.
- If the lentils have burst, turn off the heat. Add the juice of one lemon. Using a wand blender, blend everything until it is smooth.
- By now, the chicken should be cool enough to handle. Slice the chicken and wrap the slices. If you are going to be having the wraps in the next night or two, you can put these in the refrigerator. Otherwise put them in the freezer.
- To make buffalo sauce, use 1 part Tabasco to 3 parts butter. Melt the butter and whisk in the Tabasco. Put this in a small bowl, cover it, and put it in the refrigerator.
- Soften 2 tablespoons of butter. Add some chopped garlic. Place the monk fish in a casserole dish, sprinkle with salt and pepper, and brush it with the garlic butter. Cover the casserole dish and put it in the freezer.
- When the kasha is done, let it cool and then transfer to a container to put it in the refrigerator.
- Put the whole meatloaf into the refrigerator. It is much easier to slice a meatloaf when it is cold.
- Slice the assorted raw vegetables on a bias to be used like chips. Place in containers and put in the refrigerator.

Okay, so now it is Monday, dinner-on-the-go night. We're taking the wraps with us in a little cooler. Spread the Tabasco butter on the lavash or pita bread. Place chicken slices on the lavash. Add any other ingredients you would like, such as lettuce, sliced tomatoes, etc. Roll the sandwich and wrap tightly.

It's Tuesday and everyone will be home late. Before you leave in the morning, take the *frozen* crock out of the freezer, place it in the *cold* warming base, and turn it on *low*. Whoever gets home first starts some rice in the rice cooker and turns off the slow cooker. Take the roast out of the pot, and use the wand blender to puree what's left of the onions. Taste the gravy and add salt and pepper to taste. Slice the roast and serve it with some sauerkraut (prefer-

The Well-Stocked Pantry

Trying to purchase everything for a well-stocked pantry at once would make you go broke in a heartbeat. Don't look at this list and think, "She wants me to get all of that? She's crazy." Small steps: Think about acquiring items as you need them, knowing that you will be using them frequently as you cook more and more. This list is divided into sections because the pantry doesn't only refer to the dry ingredients but to all the ingredients you should have on hand to make cooking easier.

In the cupboard			
all-purpose flour	assorted beans	sugar	baking soda
whole wheat flour	assorted pasta	honey	baking powder
rice	salt	vanilla extract	assorted dried fruit
extra virgin olive oil	cider vinegar	white vinegar	red wine vinegar
balsamic vinegar	chicken stock*	beef (brown) stock*	crushed tomatoes
peeled whole tomatoes	tomato paste	anchovies	capers
arrowroot	tomato powder*	pickles	applesauce

*Recipes included in this book.

In the refrigerator			
eggs	butter	red wine	white wine
lacto-fermented veggies	miso paste	Dijon mustard	stone-ground mustard
parmesan cheese	Romano cheese	soy sauce	Worcestershire sauce

In the freezer			
space for meals	variety of meats	homemade stock	chicken pieces for stock
bones for broth	cocoa powder	variety of vegetables	bay leaves

On the spice rack			
peppercorns	garlic powder	onion powder	red pepper flakes
assorted dried peppers	celery seed	fennel seeds	cumin seeds
oregano	basil	parsley	sage
rosemary	tarragon	caraway seeds	nutmeg
allspice	cinnamon	paprika	salt

ably homemade), rice, and gravy. Save the gravy to serve with the meatloaf later in the week.

You plan on the lentil soup for Wednesday, so you take that out of the freezer on Tuesday night. We leave things to defrost on our counter. It should be thawed by morning. Put the soup in the refrigerator. When you get home, put the soup in a pot, and reheat over a low light, just until it's hot. Be careful because the soup is thick and will scorch. While the soup is heating up, get out the prepared veggies and arrange them on plates with a dollop of salted whole-milk yogurt. Once the soup is hot, taste it and add salt and pepper to taste. Don't forget to put the pickled greens on the table.

Thursday, you have a hankerin' for seafood. Get the monkfish casserole and wrapped potatoes out of the freezer and put them in the refrigerator. When you get home, check to see that the food has fully defrosted. If either is still partially frozen, pop it in the microwave for a minute or two and check on it. Put the *cold* casserole and potatoes in a *cold* oven. Heat the oven to 400°F. Once the oven comes up to 400°F, let the fish bake for 30 minutes. Remove the fish and potatoes from the oven. Put a piece of fish and a potato on each plate with some corn relish. Serve with butter and sour cream.

Friday, after a long week, you are ready for some comfort food. Meatloaf to the rescue! The meatloaf is simple: slice it cold and reheat it on a cookie sheet in a 350°F oven for about 20 minutes. Melt butter in a heavy skillet. Add the broccoli. Add about 2 tablespoons of water and cover. Melt some fat in a pot and reheat the kasha in that pot. When the water has evaporated from the broccoli, add some more butter and toss. If you saved the leftover gravy from the pot roast, you could heat that up and serve it over the kasha and meatloaf.

During the winter, we eat a lot of soup/stew meals, so we make stock "stone soup" style. Rather than putting the chicken back and neck in the freezer, I toss it into a pot with 4 or 5 quarts of filtered water and put it on the back of the stove to simmer. I also add the vegetable scraps, like carrot peels, potato peels, and celery tops, and let it all simmer on the back of the stove for a few hours. I strain out the solids, remove the meat and bones, and press what is left of the vegetables to get any liquid back into the pot. Once this is cooled, I put it in a container in the freezer and use it the next week for the stock in my meals.

Yes, it takes more effort than dialing a phone each night, but honestly, it isn't any harder than stopping at the grocery store, finding a parking spot, picking up a pre-cooked chicken and side, and standing in the checkout line behind the person with fifty items in the express lane. And if it takes another fifteen minutes a night but you don't get sick this winter, and neither does anyone else in your family, think about the time you won't be spending in doctors' offices or in bed. If you can do this for one week, you can do this for any week. Once you have formed the habit, you will feel stronger and healthier. You might find your allergies aren't as severe, or you don't get as many colds.

Epilogue

According to the archetype of the journeying hero, at some point, toward the end of the story, the hero must return home. Two things have always struck me about this part of the story. The first is that the hero must face his past, and the second is that he will be held responsible for his actions. "Home" is where I began. Thomas Wolfe said, "You can't go home again." I think, however, we all must return home, to the place where we started, or we can never really evaluate what progress we have made in our lives. Home is where I confront who I was and reconcile that person with who I am now. Home is where I come face to face with the people who know me best and find out if they respect the person I have become. And that, perhaps, is one of the most intimidating things we encounter.

We all go through phases. As a teenager, I rebelled against my parents. As an adult, I did things of which my parents did not approve, like leaving a tenured teaching job to move to Colorado for graduate school. And, as always, I returned home. I found my parents very respectful of the decision that I made to go to graduate school. I learned something very important in this: I don't need to approve of someone else's actions, but I do need to learn how to respect the person for the decisions he makes.

I take this attitude into the classroom. I firmly believe that respect is the single most lacking element in our culture. I tell my students on the first day of school that respect should be an unstated expectation, but due to many factors in our culture, I need to specifically discuss it. Many people these days have a sense of entitlement that I find disturbing. I hear how some of my students speak to their parents and to each other. They do not respect their parents, they do not respect their peers, and they do not respect themselves. If a person has no innate sense of respect for themselves, they can be easily manipulated by others, a dangerous scenario in a capitalist culture. If we are not careful, we will be raising our children to be victims of the industrialized food system. They will be manipulated into believing whatever advertisers want them to believe, which does not bode well for the future of our culture, our health, or the environment.

As I move forward, I face my past. As I learn more and more about health and nutrition, I learn to let go of any guilt that I feel about unwitting nutritional mistakes that I have made. I look forward to better decisions in the future, rather than dwelling on past errors. We used to eat conventional food. We've had phases where we got take-out or pre-fab meals at least once a week, ordering enough food to eat leftovers on another night. We never gave a second thought to the health or environmental impact our actions had. We didn't see the big picture connected to our food.

Yes, we go out to eat sometimes. Yes, we get take-out sometimes. We aren't perfectly adhering to any one set of guidelines, but we are doing a lot better now as far as eating better food—food that is better for us and better for the environment. Greg and I have learned so much about stewardship of the land—that if We The People turn our backs on the land that feeds us, We The People are going to be in big health trouble. We need to look back: How did Nature sustain itself for thousands of years before humankind tried to "tame" her? Wouldn't Nature be the best teacher?

My husband and I both work. Our two children go to public school. We have a big black dog who is afraid of lightning. We have a white picket fence. We are middle-class Americans. In many ways, we are average. Ten years ago, if someone had asked me, "What does organic mean to you?" I probably would have given some snide response deriding a granola-snacking hippie-throwback. If someone had asked me about sustainable agriculture, I probably wouldn't have said anything at all, and just given him a look of confusion. If someone would have asked me if food additives were dangerous, I would have said no.

Now I know better. I am home again, back to where all of this affects my family. The more we stick to organic fruits and vegetables, pastured meats, and raw milk from grass-fed cows, and the more we stay away from processed foods, take-out foods, and convenience foods, the better off we are. The benefits we have experienced include many fewer colds last winter, no cases of the flu, better dental checkups, much less severe seasonal allergy symptoms, and better-behaved children who are strong and definitely not suffering from obesity. Translation? Except for well visits, we didn't visit the pediatrician. We weren't running to get prescriptions filled. We didn't have to waste valuable time and energy fighting illness.

We are as busy as the next family, and we made it work. You can, too. As a friend of mine used to say, "Life is about choices." With every meal you consume, you make a choice, and that choice has consequences. If you choose to deal directly with a farmer, the food you put on your table could be sustaining the environment, fostering better health for you and your family, or working to preserve a way of life—the small family farm—that is endangered by the industrial food system. The resources are there for you, but you need to take the initiative and the responsibility. Once you take that first step, you will begin to feel a sense of empowerment about your food choices. The more steps you take, the more empowered you will become.

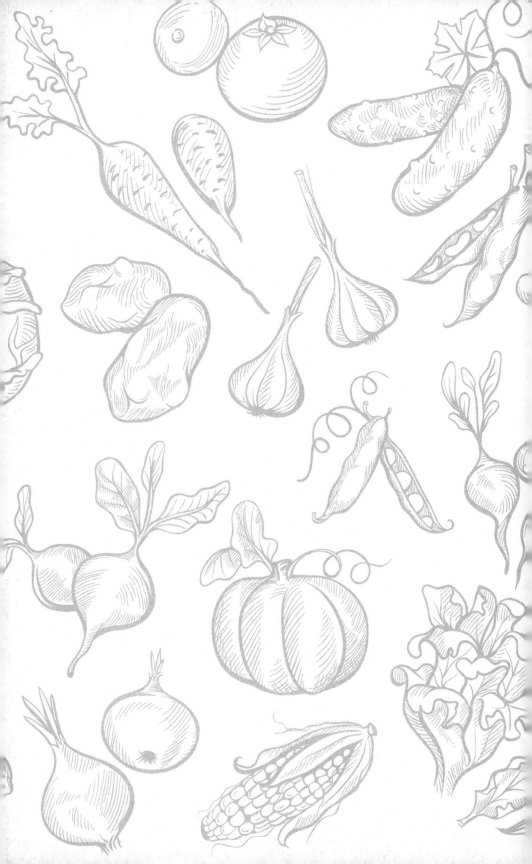

Appendix A

The Thirty-Month Plan and Why You Need One

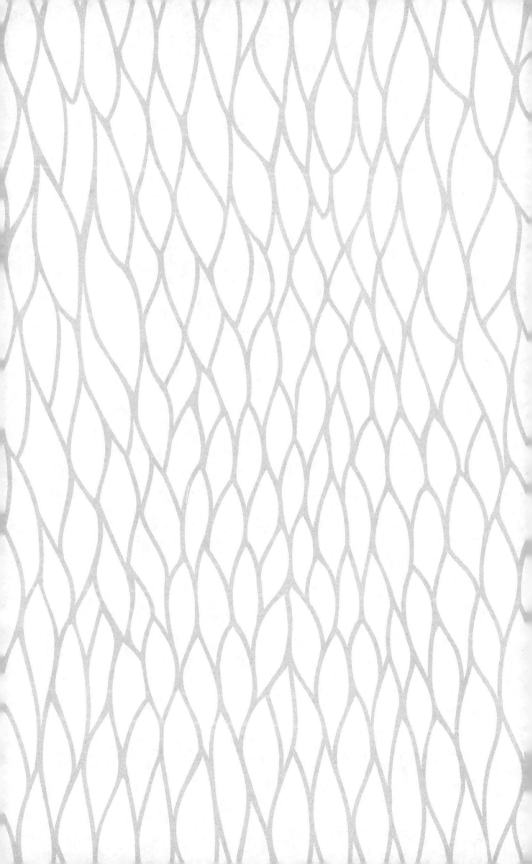

Setting goals, both long term and short term, is very important because goals give a person a sense of direction and purpose. The problem that many people encounter with goal setting is that the long-term goal looks and sounds good, but with no plan for achieving the goal, with no time limits in place, with no consideration of why the goal is important, we set ourselves up for failure. Case in point: New Year's resolutions. How many people do you know who make and break New Year's resolutions on New Year's Day?

Take a minute and ask yourself why you picked up this book: Are you feeling poorly? Concerned about your children's health and wellness? Tired of wondering what is in your food? Worried about the nutritional value of what is on your dinner table? Any of these reasons (or a gazillion others) could be the impetus for creating a Thirty-Month Plan.

Next, make a decision about something you want to achieve; it could be anything, food-related or not. You can choose something like changing the way you eat, keeping your house clean, or writing a book, just as long as you have a clear path to achievement.

The key to success is making a plan. One of the drawbacks of our GPS-guided society is that people can no longer read a map. Knowing how to read a map and planning a route to get from point A to point B is an important life skill. It translates into how we travel through our lives: can you plan a route? Can you see alternate routes? If there is a roadblock, can you find a way around it, or do you depend upon a GPS? A computer can't do all your thinking and planning for you. Life is an epic, an *Odyssey*, and we learn through trial and error how to navigate it.

As I have been emphasizing all along, don't try to make huge changes all at once. I'll use our experiences gardening as an illustration. Greg and I had a twenty-five-by-twenty-five-foot garden our first year in our house. We produced a lot of tomatoes, lettuces, cucumbers, and several varieties of peppers. This was before children, and I had the time necessary to maintain the garden. Once the kids came along, things got more difficult and the gardens were not as successful. Oh, we had good years with beans or cucumbers, but nothing like the success we had the first year. We eventually scaled back and had much more success by using one-and-a-half-by-twenty-foot border gardens where I planted edibles instead of flowers. Sometimes less is more.

I do not recommend doing any of the planning I am about to explain on a computer or any other electronic device. No one will be grading your penmanship. No one will be taking off points for neatness. The problem with a computer is the limitation of the screen. For working on a book, it's great; I can only see so much of what I am writing at a time, and that keeps me focused on the task at hand. When working on a Thirty-Month Plan, however, you need to see the big picture, the entire thing at once. Use a pencil and a piece of paper and be prepared to erase as things change. Sometimes opportunities arise that change our direction or maybe give us the chance to complete a task before we thought we would be able to do so. However, you must commit your plan to writing. You can have a lot of amorphous ideas in your head, but they don't mean anything until you can communicate them to others. When we commit things to writing we make the ideas part of our concrete world because we can see them. As an English teacher of over twenty years, I have come to see that much of my students' anxiety about writing comes from this stage of transforming the abstract into the concrete, where it will be on paper and they have to keep looking at it. Even if your goal is something as simple and succinct as, "I will only eat restaurant food once a month," you need to write it down so you are forced to keep looking at it.

If you are creating a Thirty-Month Plan for your family, call a family meeting and get everyone's input. Your family will not invest in a project if they were not part of the planning process. If the plan is for you, then find a quiet place and time to really consider what it is that you want for yourself. Remember, not pie in the sky, but something simple. You picked up this book, so I will assume that taking control of what is on your table is a goal of yours, and I will use that as my example plan.

Create a grid on a piece of paper, three columns by ten rows. Label each rectangle with a month and year or months 1–30:

Month 1 _____	Month 2 _____	Month 3 _____
Month 4 _____	Month 5 _____	Month 6 _____
Month 7 _____	Month 8 _____	Month 9 _____
Month 10 _____	Month 11 _____	Month 12 _____
Month 13 _____	Month 14 _____	Month 15 _____
Month 16 _____	Month 17 _____	Month 18 _____
Month 19 _____	Month 20 _____	Month 21 _____
Month 22 _____	Month 23 _____	Month 24 _____

YEAR 1 (Months 1–12)
YEAR 2 (Months 13–24)

YEAR 3	Month 25 _____	Month 26 _____	Month 27 _____
	Month 28 _____	Month 29 _____	Month 30 _____ Eating 90 percent organic foods

Put your end goal in the last box.

Look at the end goal. Consider where you are at present and think of one small thing that you can do, right now, that would start you on the journey to achieving that goal. If you are in the fast food rut, and you want to break that cycle and become someone who eats healthier food that is better for both you and the environment, then a Thirty-Month Plan to eat food that is mostly produced organically is a great goal. So what is one thing, one small thing, that you can do immediately, that won't turn your world completely upside-down?

Write that in the first rectangle:

YEAR 1	Month 1 _____ Limit eating fast food to once a day	Month 2 _____	Month 3 _____
	Month 4 _____	Month 5 _____	Month 6 _____
	Month 7 _____	Month 8 _____	Month 9 _____
	Month 10 _____	Month 11 _____	Month 12 _____
YEAR 2	Month 13 _____	Month 14 _____	Month 15 _____
	Month 16 _____	Month 17 _____	Month 18 _____
	Month 19 _____	Month 20 _____	Month 21 _____
	Month 22 _____	Month 23 _____	Month 24 _____

YEAR 3	Month 25 _____	Month 26 _____	Month 27 _____
	Month 28 _____	Month 29 _____	Month 30 _____ Eating 90 percent organic foods

These are good starting and ending points. That first goal is a small, doable step. Notice it doesn't say "stop eating fast food." That would mean an entire change in lifestyle overnight, and those kinds of changes rarely hold up for too long. So, in the first month, the only thing you would focus on is not eating fast food for more than one meal a day. Technically, if you only eat once a day, you can still achieve this goal and still eat nothing but fast food. But that aside, if you are the kind of person who stops at a donut place for a coffee and a sandwich for breakfast, gets pizza for lunch, and then stops at a restaurant chain for "Curbside Service" for dinner, the one change of eating breakfast at home, or packing a lunch to take to work, can be a difficult goal to achieve. Keep in mind that it takes a few weeks to develop or break a habit. By focusing on that one small change, you have a better chance of developing the new habit. If the first month's goal was something bigger, like cutting out fast food entirely, you may find yourself completely overwhelmed and give up after two or three days.

Next you need to pencil in the route you *think* you might take:

YEAR 1	Month 1 _____ Limit eating fast food to once a day	Month 2 _____ No fast food burgers and fries for lunch	Month 3 _____ Make dinner from scratch three times a week
	Month 4 _____ Shop only around the perimeter of the grocery store two weeks	Month 5 _____ Plan menus for dinner on a weekly basis	Month 6 _____ Research community supported agriculture
	Month 7 _____ Make lunches at home	Month 8 _____ Research sources for eggs and meat	Month 9 _____ *Assess budget to purchase freezer*
	Month 10 _____	Month 11 _____ Read a book on food preservation	Month 12 _____

YEAR 2	Month 13 _____ Learn how to can	Month 14 _____ Can spaghetti sauce	Month 15 _____ Bake bread for lunches
	Month 16 _____	Month 17 _____ Make a pumpkin pie from scratch (no cans)	Month 18 _____ *Join a CSA Farm*
	Month 19 _____	Month 20 _____	Month 21 _____
	Month 22 _____	Month 23 _____ Plant two tomato plants in pots	Month 24 _____
YEAR 3	Month 25 _____	Month 26 _____	Month 27 _____
	Month 28 _____	Month 29 _____	Month 30 _____ Eating 90 percent organic foods

Notice there are blanks. Sometimes you can't see the step for that month, but like all things that grow organically, what you need to do will come naturally based upon what has happened in the months prior. Just remember to keep looking at the plan, with a pencil in your hand, and update and revise as things happen. Notice in the Month 6 block, it says, "Research community supported agriculture," but it doesn't say "Join a CSA Farm" until Month 18. Why wait a year? Why not join a CSA farm immediately? As the CSA movement is gaining momentum, many farms have a "Wait List" for families to join them. So when you know for sure you can join the CSA, you would fill that into the block.

The italic print indicates revisions to the initial plan. Month 8 is the month to research sources for pastured eggs and meat. Month 9 has a revision. Initially, Month 9 was the month to begin baking homemade bread for lunch sandwiches. After doing the research, you realized that you need to save money to purchase a freezer in order to buy meat in bulk and store it. Bread baking gets pushed back to Month 15, and an analysis of the budget moves to the forefront.

Also notice what some of the goals are—not all of them are lofty or difficult, nor would they take all month. Month 17's goal of making a pumpkin pie from scratch doesn't sound all that difficult, but if you have never made a pie crust, let alone baked off a pumpkin and made puree, it can seem rather intimidating. But what a wonderful thing to put on the table next Thanksgiving dinner: from farm to table, from pumpkin patch to pie!

Why all of the copies of the chart? If you were looking at the last chart only, you wouldn't have taken that moment to consider just an end point and then just a starting point. Our culture overwhelms us with ideas and images, which is counterproductive to our ability to focus. Our culture shows us images of end results—the dieter's image before and after the crash diet—but does not consider the process that led up to the first image, what happened after the second image was taken, nor what the process was that got the person from fat to thin.

Your Thirty-Month Plan can be multifaceted. My personal Thirty-Month Plan includes things like finishing this book and making a good blueberry jam. As months pass, if I have achieved that month's goal, I get a sticker in the box. If I don't achieve the goal, I just cross out or erase and move the goal to the next month, or maybe even a couple of months away. You must be flexible enough to see that Plan A may not work the way you thought and that you need to take other steps in order to achieve that particular goal. You can include your food goals and your career goals, your fitness goals and your emotional goals. The plan will work for any aspect of your life because while goal setting creates a purpose for your actions, achieving the small steps toward the big goal creates confidence. When I have months where the goal wasn't met, I sit down and assess why and then go about revising.

I can't creep into your head and figure out what you need to do, and neither can anyone else. Beware the many people out there being prescriptive, telling you what you need to do. This illustrates a larger cultural problem: we have stopped thinking for ourselves. We let big corporations think for us, when their primary interest is money, not the health and well-being of the general population. Food empowerment begins with self-empowerment. Stop listening to commercials, infomercials, and corporate-sponsored reports, and listen to your heart. You know yourself better than I know you, and this is why I can't outline a one-size-fits-all plan. I can only make suggestions. Just take your time and follow your instincts.

Any time anyone contemplates a life change, there should be serious self-evaluation. As we all know, only rarely do people make drastic lifestyle changes that stick. The best and most permanent changes are those that occur organically. You may find that you are having trouble with a month's goal and want to continue to focus on that one thing for a couple of months. Once that change becomes "normal," you can evaluate how and what to change next. Then pick up your pencil and revise the plan.

Sometimes you will have external factors that prevent you from working toward your goal: work gets hectic, your son gets sick with the flu and can't kick it, you break your ankle. These things may force you to change your plan. That is why I use pencil. Many things happen that will send you down a road you weren't planning to take. But don't let any of these things prevent you from continuing to work toward that last rectangle. I never forget to reward myself. The first time I was hunting for stickers, my daughter (who had hoarded them all in her desk drawer) laughed at me: "Really, Mommy? You need a sticker for your own paper?" Yes. Yes, I did. And I am still proud of that first sticker on my paper.

Appendix B

Food Preservation and Recipes

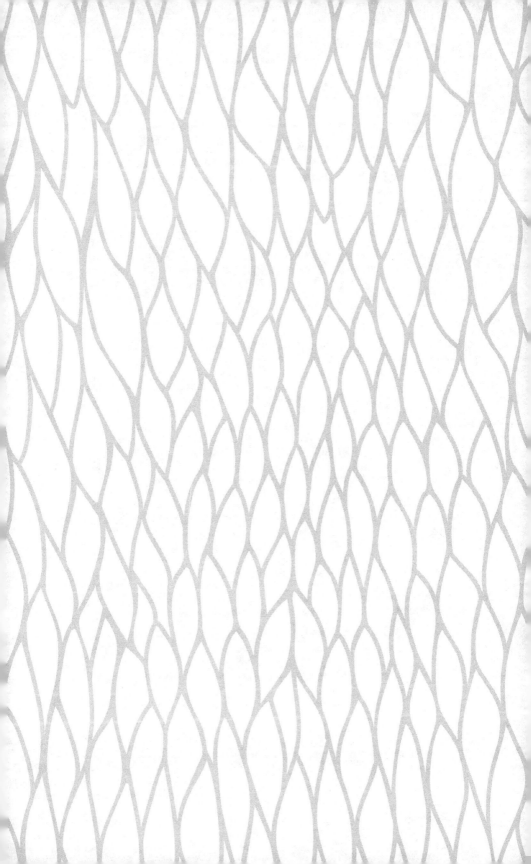

What follows here are recipes and instructions that I have gleaned over the years. There are two resources to which I continually return: *The Philadelphia Public Schools Lessons in Elementary Domestic Science*, a textbook that belonged to my grandmother, and *Mrs. Owens' Cook Book & Useful Hints for the Household*, circa 1883. I have adapted the recipes for the modern cook because Mrs. Owen's recipes say things like, "Place meat in a dripping pan and place it in a hot oven until done." That isn't really much to go on. But what that does tell me is that I should put the meat in a rack inside the pan so juices can collect underneath.

Lacto-Fermentation Recipes

General Brine I: (if you have whey available)
1 cup filtered water
1 tablespoon unrefined sea salt
¼ cup whey*

Mix together until the salt is dissolved.

---

* People who are lactose intolerant can sometimes tolerate whey; but those with casein allergies should avoid it.

General Brine II:*
1 cup filtered water
2 tablespoons
    unrefined sea salt
Mix together until the
    salt is dissolved.

Sour Pickle Spears
3–4 kirby cucumbers
1 large dill flower (or 1
    teaspoon dill seed)
2 cloves of garlic
horseradish or grape
    leaves (optional,
    but recommended)
1 cup filtered water
2 tablespoons sea salt

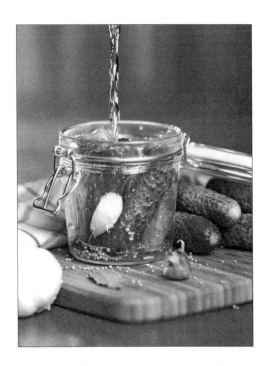

Dissolve the salt in the water. Cut the cucumbers into spears. If you are using horseradish or grape leaves (which help the cucumbers retain crispness), place them in the bottom of the jar. Add dill and garlic. Arrange the cucumber spears vertically in a wide mouth canning jar. Cover with the salt water. If the solution doesn't cover the tops of the cucumbers, add enough water to cover. Close the lid tightly. Leave in a warm spot for 2–3 days. You should see tiny bubbles starting to form in the brine. Move to cold storage.

Cellar Salad
2 medium turnips, quartered and sliced thinly or grated
2 medium beets, quartered and sliced thinly or grated
1 small onion, sliced thinly
1 medium carrot, grated
1 small head of cabbage, cored and shredded

---

* If no whey is available or when preparing food for someone who is dairy-free.

1 tablespoon unrefined sea salt
1/4 cup whey (or use an additional 1 tablespoon
    of unrefined sea salt)

In a large bowl, mix all of the ingredients except the whey. If you are not using whey, use both tablespoons of salt. Cover with a tea towel or a plate and let stand for 30 minutes. The salt should have drawn out a lot of moisture from the vegetables. If you are using whey, add it now and mix thoroughly. Pack the mixture into a clean wide-mouth canning jar and cover tightly. Leave in a warm spot for 2–3 days. Transfer to cold storage. Do not over-pack the jar as this mixture tends to grow!

Odds-n-Ends Salad

You can use whatever you have on hand, really. One day I found five grape tomatoes sitting on the counter. What was I supposed to do with five grape tomatoes that needed to be used before they were fodder for the compost heap? I poked around the fridge and threw together a bunch of odds-n-ends. Now, when the sweet corn comes in, we always cook an extra couple of ears so we can have more of this salad.

Corn kernels from two ears of corn (cooked)
Grape tomatoes, quartered
1 sweet pepper, small dice
1 jalapeño (or other pepper, hot or not) sliced
1/2 bunch chopped cilantro
2 green onions, thinly sliced

In a large bowl, mix all of the ingredients. Pack the mixture into a clean wide-mouth canning jar. Add enough general brine to cover and cover the jar tightly. Leave in a warm spot for 2–3 days. Transfer to cold storage.

Dehydrating Recipes

Apple Rings
Peel and core the apples. Cut crosswise to make rings. Place on the dehydrator in a single layer. After 10–12 hours, test for doneness. The rings should be dry but slightly pliable. Store in a cool cupboard in a tightly sealed jar.

Blueberries
I live in New Jersey, one of the blueberry capitals of the world. We pick them at a local blueberry farm and freeze and dry them until

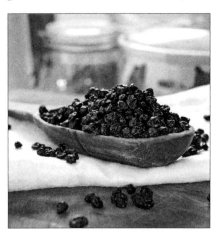

the season is over.

Wash the blueberries and leave them to dry in a single layer on a towel. Once they are dry, transfer them to the dehydrator, making sure that they are not too close together to ensure good air circulation. They will look and feel like raisins when they are done. Store in a cool cupboard in a tightly sealed jar.

Tomato Powder
I can a lot of tomatoes, but at the end of the season, it doesn't seem practical to go through all of the hassle of canning for one or two quarts of tomatoes. Instead, I make tomato powder that can be added directly to spaghetti sauce to thicken it, or mixed with water and used like tomato paste.

Wash the tomatoes. Slice in half and scoop out the seeds. Place in the dehydrator. Dry them until they are hard as a rock. Break up the pieces and put them in a blender or food processor. Process until it is a very fine powder. Store in a tightly sealed jar.

Fruit Leather

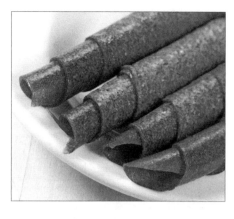

You must get the special trays for making leather. Anything I tried to rig up resulted in an abysmal failure.

In a blender, combine 1 cup of applesauce and one cup of berries. Blend until everything is very smooth. Pour onto a greased leather tray and dry until it sets (about 7–8 hours). Flip it over and continue to dry until it is leathery. Put it on a piece of baking parchment and roll it up. I store this in a bail-top "spaghetti" canister. I have replaced the berries with sour cherries, cut-up super-ripe peaches, and cut-up super-ripe plums. This is a great way to use up fruit that is about to become a fruit fly factory. If it has already become a fruit fly factory, it is too late!

Canning Recipes

For the past few years, I have entered my canned goods in the Burlington County Farm Fair and Middletown Grange Fair and have racked up a few ribbons. Here are some of my blue ribbon recipes.

Sweet Tomato Jam

4–5 pounds tomatoes, peeled
4–6 chili peppers, deseeded and sliced thin (amount depends upon how hot you want to make this)
1 1/2-inch piece of ginger root, grated
1 medium head of garlic, peeled and chopped
3 lemons, zested and juiced
1 small shallot, minced
4 cups sugar

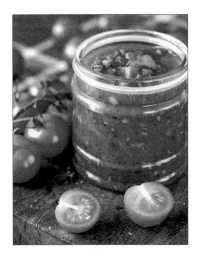

Chop the tomatoes and transfer juice and all into a large non-reactive pot. Add the remaining ingredients, and stir until the sugar has dissolved. When it starts to simmer, turn the heat up to boil off the excess water. Continue cooking until the mixture turns translucent (this could take up to 3 hours). The jam tends to stick, so stirring regularly is necessary and constant stirring is required at the end of the cooking process. Ladle hot jam into hot jars and process. Leave jam to rest for at least 1 month before eating. This pairs very nicely with goat cheese, and makes a wonderful glaze for pork or chicken.

Salsa Inspired by Rosemary's recipe
10 quarts of tomatoes, peeled and chopped
2 large onions, chopped
1/2 cup salt

Mix these together in a colander, and let drain for 3 hours. Transfer to a non-reactive pot. Then add:

2 stalks celery, sliced
2 green onions, chopped
1–2 jalapeños, sliced (deseed for less heat)
1–2 green chilies (deseed for less heat)
1 cup sugar
1 cup vinegar
12 ounces tomato paste

Simmer for 20 minutes. Pack in hot pint jars and process 20 minutes.

Grape Jelly

3 lbs. of grapes, washed and stemmed
1/2 cup water
7 cups sugar
1 pouch liquid pectin

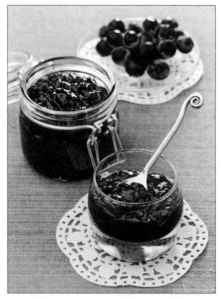

Place grapes in a large pot with the water and bring to a simmer. Simmer for 5–10 minutes. Crush the grapes with a potato masher or long-handled meat tenderizer (I use the plunger from my grinder), and simmer another 5–10 minutes. Strain juice through a jelly bag (see note below). Do not squeeze the bag! In a clean pot, measure 4 cups of the prepared juice. Stir in the sugar. Do not reduce the sugar if you are using standard pectin! If you want to reduce the sugar, use pectin made especially for low-sugar recipes. Bring the mixture to a full rolling boil—a boil that cannot be stirred down. Quickly stir in the pectin and return to a full rolling boil. Boil for exactly 1 minute. Turn off heat and let stand for 1 minute. Skim any foam from the top. Ladle into prepared jars and process.

Note: I used an old sheet and made jelly bags that fit inside my chinois. When I am done, I can throw the jelly bag in the washer and it gets completely clean—no pulp hanging on anywhere.

You can do a "second pressing" to make another batch of jelly: Return the pulp to the pot, and add 1/2 cup of water. Bring up to a simmer and return it to the jelly bag. This time you can squeeze the bag to get all of the juice out of it. The result will taste great, but it will be a little cloudy.

Odd Animal Parts

Heart Stew

1 veal heart, cleaned of tendons or anything squishy—leave just
   dense meat
1 pound veal stew meat
1 slice of bacon
2 medium onions, chopped
2 whole cloves
1 pint beef stock
2 teaspoons sugar
salt and pepper

Cut the heart into bite-sized pieces and place in a brine of 1
cup of water, 1 teaspoon of sugar, 1 teaspoon of salt, and 1 clove.
Leave in the refrigerator for 10 hours. Drain the heart pieces. Make
more brine and add the heart. Let sit overnight in the refrigerator.
In the morning, drain the pieces. Heat the oven to 250°F. On the
stovetop, render the fat out of the bacon in a large Dutch oven

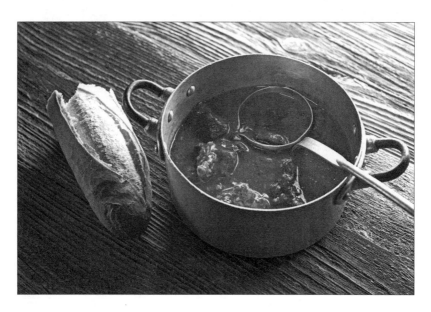

or other heavy-bottomed pot that can go into your oven. Remove the bacon, crumble, and set aside. Add the onions and cook in the bacon fat until they begin to caramelize (turn golden brown). Add the stock and scrape up any bits that are sticking to the bottom of the pot. Turn off the heat. Add the stew meat and the heart pieces. Put the lid on and put the whole thing into the preheated oven. Let this cook for 3 hours. Remove from the oven. Everything should be very tender. The gravy can be thickened by adding some cream and stirring it through over a low heat on the stove top.

Liver that Natalie Can Eat

From the title of this recipe, you probably figured out that I am not a fan of liver and onions. But I was always a fan of my grandmother's chopped liver, so here's the concoction of Greg's that I love.

1 1/2 pounds sliced beef liver, cut into strips
1 large onion, chopped
salt
chicken fat (schmaltz) for frying
2 hardboiled eggs, chopped

Heat the schmaltz in a heavy skillet and fry the onions until they are transparent and cooked through. Remove them from the pan. Add some more schmaltz and add the liver in a single layer. Do this in batches if necessary. Turn the liver so it browns on two sides. Once all of the liver is cooked, put it in the bowl of a food processor with the onions and pulse until everything is chopped, but not smooth. Remove the liver from the processor and mix in the eggs. Add salt and pepper to taste.

Resources

Websites

Agrilicious
www.agrilicious.org
Allows you to set up a local "neighborhood" to help put you in contact with local farmers. The listings are comprehensive and growing.

Eat Wild
www.eatwild.com
Great information about grass-fed foods and an extremely comprehensive listing of farms by state. This website was a gateway for us!

Local Harvest
www.localharvest.org
Contains links to help you find farmer's markets and CSAs in your area. I have found it very easy to navigate.

Sustainable Table
www.sustainabletable.org
Includes lots of good information about sustainable practice. The shopping guides and shop sustainable menus are especially helpful if you are just getting started trying to find foods that are in season.

The Weston A. Price Foundation
www.westonaprice.org
An amazing archive of articles about nutrition and health written by a variety of authors about technical issues that are put into layman's terms.

Books

Nutrition and Physical Degeneration, Weston A. Price
This book is an incredible study of indigenous populations that compares traditional diets to "modern" refined foods diets. The research is a bit dated, but the case Dr. Price makes is compelling. Due to the introduction of Western-style eating almost all over the globe, it would be impossible to try to replicate his research today. I feel it is irresponsible for Dr. Price's research to be so readily dismissed because of its age. While Nathan Pritikin proposed a radically different diet, he was suggesting the same idea: We wouldn't have so much disease if we ate more nutritious food!

The Unhealthy Truth, Robyn O'Brien
Part of what is so very important about this book is that Robyn O'Brien does not pretend to be anything but what she is: a mom with children who were not 100 percent healthy, who tried to solve the mystery of their ailments. Her journey and the information she imparts are extremely important for all concerned parents.

Nourishing Traditions, Sally Fallon
This is much more than a cookbook! In addition to amazing recipes, this book includes a lot of valuable information about nutrition and health. There are sidebars all throughout the cookbook with quotes from other authors that supplement the information in the chapter. My husband and I have a lot of fun with "Know Your Ingredients"!

Everything I Want to Do Is Illegal, Joel Salatin
Most of us do not give a thought to the power of some of our government agencies. We don't think about what creates food safety, or the factors that lead to the production of food unsafe for human consumption. This book explains both from the farmer's perspective, a voice that needs to be heard but thus far has not been given the attention it deserves. As non-farmers, most of us have no idea the implications of the regulations regarding food production. This book explains all of that and more.

The American Way of Eating, Tracie McMillan

This book takes the reader on an "insider's" tour of three aspects of the food industry—commercial farming, retail, and restaurant. The narrative nature makes for fluid reading and it is very informative for the uninitiated.

Long Way on a Little: An Earth Lover's Companion for Enjoying Meat, Pinching Pennies and Living Deliciously, Shannon Hayes

This is a cookbook plus so much more. For someone beginning the journey toward better food, or someone who is already on the road, *Long Way on a Little* is chock full of advice about cooking foods with which you may not be familiar.

Spices

Penzeys Spices

www.penzeys.com

We have been very happy with the quality of the spices we purchase from Penzeys. They have great variety and the prices are competitive.

Frontier Co-op

www.frontiercoop.com

Another great source for spices and much more. They also have a great variety of teas and other products.

Selected Bibliography

Armson, Myra. "Gas Mixtures Help Preserve the Quality of Packaged Meats." *Scientist Live*, April 1, 2013, http://www.scientistlive.com/content/23480 (accessed September 9, 2014).

Bernstein, Zachary. "Public Health Experts Warn Next Generation May Have Shorter Life Span as a Result of Obesity." *ThinkProgress*, May 4, 2012, http://thinkprogress.org/health/2012/05/04/478249/obesity-life-expectency/ (accessed September 9, 2014).

Christie, Chris. "Governor's Fiscal Year 2013 Budget." New Jersey State Office of Management and Budget, 2012, http://www.state.nj.us/treasury/omb.

Cohen, Robert. "Homogenized Milk: Rocket Fuel for Cancer." Health 101, http://health101.org/art_milk_cancer_fuel.htm.

Cone, Marla. "New Study: Autism Linked to Environment." *Scientific American*, January 9, 2009, http://www.scientificamerican.com/article/autism-rise-driven-by-environment/ (accessed September 9, 2013).

Curb, David, Gilbert Wergowske, Joan C. Dobbs, Robert D. Abbott, and Boji Huang. "Serum Lipid Effects of a High–Monounsaturated Fat Diet Based on Macadamia Nuts." *Archives of Internal Medicine* 160, no. 8 (2000): 1154–58, http://archinte.ama-assn.org/cgi/reprint/160/8/1154.pdf (accessed July 22, 2010).

Eicher, Annie. "A Glossary of Terms for Farmers and Gardeners." *Organic Agriculture: Michigan Conservation Districts*, July 10, 2010.

Eng, Monica. "Pesticides in Your Peaches: Tribune and USDA Studies Find Pesticides, Some in Excess of EPA Rules, in the Fragrant Fruit." *Chicago Tribune*, August 12, 2009, http://www.chicagotribune.com/lifestyles /health/chi-0812-peaches-pesticides_mainaug12-story.html#page=1 (accessed September 18, 2014).

Flegal, Katherine, Margaret Carroll, Cynthia Ogden, and Lester Ogden. "Prevalence and Trends in Obesity Among US Adults, 1999–2008." *JAMA & Archives* 303, no. 3 (2010): 235–41, http://jama.ama-assn.org /cgi/content/full/303/3/235?ijkey=ijKHq6YbJn3Oo&keytype=ref&sit eid=amajnls (accessed July 7, 2010).

Forristal, Linda. "The Murky World of High-Fructose Corn Syrup." *Wise Traditions*, December 3, 2003, http://www.westonaprice.org/health -topics/the-murky-world-of-high-fructose-corn-syrup/ (January 11, 2013).

Immuno Laboratories, Inc. "Overweight and Obesity in Children." *Better Health USA*, July 10, 2010, http://www.betterhealthusa.com /public/227.cfm.

James, Walene. *Immunization: The Reality Behind The Myth.* Westport, CT: Bergen & Garvey, 1995.

"Maps of Trends in Diagnosed Diabetes and Obesity." Centers for Disease Control and Prevention, 2011, http://www.cdc.gov/diabetes/statistics.

McAvoy, Miles. "Genetically Modified Organisms." USDA Organic policy memorandum, April 15, 2011, http://www.ams.usda.gov/AMSv1.0/get file?dDocName=STELPRDC5090396 (accessed August 22, 2014).

McNamara, Melissa. "Diet Industry is Big Business." CBS News, December 1, 2006, http://www.cbsnews.com/news/diet-industry-is-big-business / (accessed January 11, 2013).

Monte, Tom. "All About Pritikin." Pritikin Longevity Center, July 7, 2010, http://www.pritikin.com/index.php?option=com_content&view=articl e&id=61&Itemid=89.

National Institute of Food and Agriculture. Agriculture and Food Research Initiative—Foundational Program. http://www.nifa.usda.gov/funding /afri/afri.html.

Pfeiffer, Sacha, with Dan Charles. "U.S. Organic Board Bans Use of Antibiotic 'Streptomycin.'" *Here & Now*. Boston NPR. May 2, 2014.

Philpott, Tom. "How GMOs Unleashed a Pesticide Gusher." *Mother Jones*, October 3, 2012., http://www.motherjones.com/tom-philpott/2012/10/how-gmos-ramped-us-pesticide-use (accessed August 22, 2014).

Price, Weston. *Nutrition and Physical Degeneration*. LaMesa, California: Price-Pottenger Nutritional Foundation, 2009. Originally New York: P. B. Hoeber, 1939.

Simpoulos, A. P. "The Importance of the Ratio of Omega-6/Omega-3 Essential Fatty Acids." *Biomedicine and Pharmacotherapy* 56, no. 8 (October 2002): 365–79, http://www.ncbi.nlm.nih.gov/pubmed/12442909.

Siri-Tarino, Patty, Qi Sun, Frank B. Hu, and Ronald M. Krauss. "Meta-analysis of Prospective Cohort Studies Evaluating the Association of Saturated Fat with Cardiovascular Disease." *American Journal of Clinical Nutrition* 91, no. 3 (2010): 535–46, www.ajcn.org/cgi/content/abstract/91/3/535.

Vital Statistics of the United States, 1900–1970, U.S. Public Health Service, annual, Vol. I and Vol. II; 1971–2001, U.S. National Center for Health Statistics, *Vital Statistics of the United States*, annual; *National Vital Statistics Report (NVSR)* (formerly *Monthly Vital Statistics Report*); and unpublished data.

Williams, Rachel. "Many Parents Failing to Read to Children, Survey Shows." *Guardian*, April 29, 2010, http://www.guardian.co.uk/education/2010/apr/30/children-parents-reading-stories (accessed January 2013).

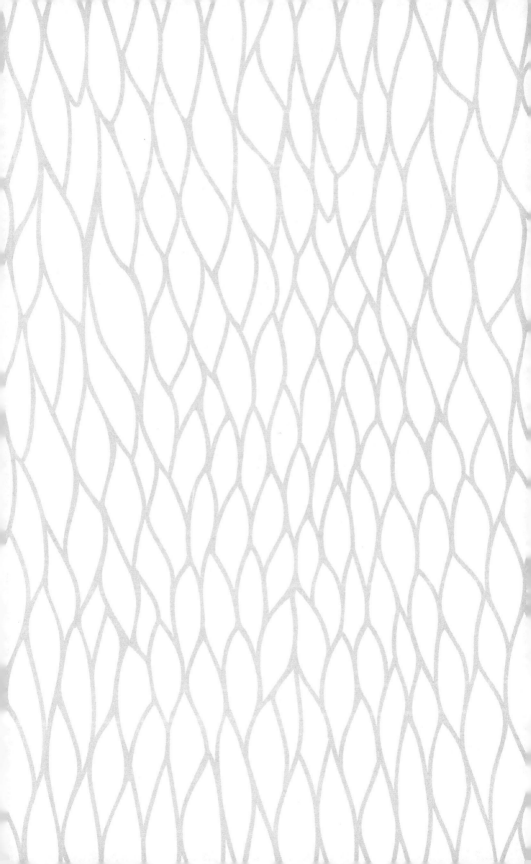

Index

all-natural, 46
antibiotics, 23, 45, 59, 60, 61–62
apples, 34, 44, 46, 59, 93,
    120, 156
applesauce, 120, 121, 133, 157
Atkins diet, 19, 26

biodiversity, 46–47, 88
biodynamic, 87, 88
blueberries, 121, 149, 156
bones, 74, 115–18, 134, 135
brine, 49–51, 153–54

canning, 7, 115–120, 121–23,
    157–59
cancer, 9, 10, 42
capitalism, 26, 41, 53, 66, 138
carbohydrates, 18, 19, 20, 44, 104
cellar salad, 154–55
cheese, 5, 20, 44, 52, 64, 78,
    81, 82
chemical fertilizers, 88, 89, 90
community supported agriculture
    (CSA), 75–76, 79, 99,
    101, 105, 147, 148
concentrated animal feeding
    operations (CAFOs), 58,
    61–62, 75, 90, 91

consumerism, 7, 32, 53
convenience foods, 7, 10, 33, 35,
    41, 51–52, 102, 139
cooking
    as a family activity, 36,
        108–9, 120, 121
    for beginners, 99–100, 101,
        109, 122, 123
    from scratch, 9, 10, 99, 122,
        127–36
    kitchen equipment, 108, 114,
        130
    meal planning, 99, 101,
        113–114, 127–36
costs
    CSAs, 76
    equipment, 75, 119, 120
    farmer-direct vs.
        supermarkets, 74–76, 94
    take-out, 105
    whole foods vs. processed,
        44, 121
crop rotation, 89–90
culture of busy, 6–7, 31–34,
    78, 139

dairy, 58, 60–61. *See also* milk
dehydrating, 120–21, 156–57

Demeter USA, 88
diabetes, 7, 20, 42, 66
diet industry. *See also* specific
    diet programs
    body image and, 15–16, 17
    connection to processed
        foods, 16–17, 18–20, 24
    failures of, 17–19, 36, 149
    fat and, 8, 19–20, 23

eggs, 26, 43, 78–79
    conventional, 58, 59–60
essential oils, 22

family dinners,
    decline of, 31, 34, 36
    importance, 5–6 , , 34
family farms. *See* small farms
fast food, 16–17, 23, 26, 33, 34,
    91, 103, 146–47
fat
    anti-fat movement, 18–20,
        23, 65
    as a moral issue, 7–8
    importance of, 23, 91
    refined foods and, 8, 65
    rendering, 21–22
feedlots. *See* concentrated animal
    feeding operations
    (CAFOs)
Food and Drug Administration
    (FDA), 41, 46, 59, 80
food industry, 7–8, 9–10
    global food model, 33,
        43–44, 58–59
    government and, 41–42
food marketing, 18, 20, 21, 23,
    41, 44–45, 52–53, 138
fruit leather, 157

gardening, 118, 144
genetically modified organisms
    (GMOs), 46–48, 60, 89
glyphosate, 48. *See also* pesticides
grape jelly, 159
Great Depression, 9
Greek-style yogurt, 35–36

heart disease, 7, 23
heart stew, 160–61
Hebrew school, 5
high-fructose corn syrup, 19, 42,
    47, 48

industrial agriculture,
    rise of, 7, 10
    problems with, 47, 83. *See*
        also concentrated animal
        feeding operations,
        pesticides

kosher, 5

lacto-fermentation, 35, 49–51,
    153–55
Liver that Natalie Can Eat, 161
local food, 33, 46, 59, 76–77,
    93, 162

meal planning, 100, 101–2,
    103–5, 122–23, 128–36.
    See also under cooking
meat
    beef, 58, 90–91
    chickens, 58, 91–92
    conventional, 75, 90
    fish, 58, 63–64
    free-range, 91–92
    grass-fed, 63, 90

grass-finished, 90
organ, 92, 160–61
pasture-raised, 60, 62, 73,
    74–75, 90–92, 139, 148
veal, 62
milk
    grass-fed, 36, 79–80, 90, 139
    pasteurized, 35, 64–66
    raw. *See* raw milk
monocultures, 46–47, 48,
    88–89, 90

National Organics Standards
    Board, 59
Nature's Sunlight Farm, 73,
    77–78, 79, 81–82, 94
Nolt, Mark and Maryann. *See*
    Nature's Sunlight Farm

obesity
    as a symptom, 23–24
    childhood, 9, 20, 34, 42, 139
    rise in, 8–9, 16, 17, 42, 47, 52
Odds-n-Ends Salad, 155
organic
    certification label, 46, 59, 93
    definition, 45–46, 48, 87–89
    farming, 48, 89
    food, 36, 45–46, 74, 76,
        139, 146

pantry stocking, 101, 103–4,
    106, 108, 122–23, 133–34
peaches, 24, 59, 120, 121, 157
pesticides, 45–46, 48, 59, 88, 90
pickling, 48, 49, 106, 120,
    121, 154
Price, Weston A., 25, 163

Pritikin Diet, 17–18, 20, 23
Pritikin, Nathan, 17–18, 19–20,
    26, 163
Pritikin Promise, The (Pritikin),
    18, 26
processed foods
    addictiveness of, 33, 52
    convenience of, 33, 51, 64, 66
    definition, 48, 51–52
    health issues related to, 7, 8,
        23, 42–43, 51
    loss of nutrients in, 25,
        51–52, 64–65
protein, 18, 19, 25, 26, 42, 62,
    64, 65–66

raw milk
    benefits of, 139
    legality of, 66, 79–80
    safety of, 80–81
    taste of, 78, 79, 80
    uses for, 35
recombinant bovine growth
    hormone (rBGH), 60, 67
refined
    carbohydrates, 20
    foods, 8, 20, 23, 25, 33, 42,
        48, 51–52, 64, 66, 163
    grains, 19, 42, 104
    sugars, 19, 24–25, 42
Robinson, Jo, 73–74

Salatin, Joel, 81–82, 95, 163
Salsa Inspired by Rosemary, 158
Simple Sautéed Chicken, 107–8
Sisyphus, 7
small farms
    buying from, 74–75, 76–77,
        93–94

costs. *See under* costs, famer-
    direct vs. supermarket
decline of, 7, 94
farmer-consumer
    relationships, 76–77,
    82–83
how to locate, 73–74
mutual accountability,
    80–81, 83
snacking, 8, 35, 121
social media, 32, 36
soup, 74, 106, 113, 115–18, 119,
    120–21, 128, 131,
    134–35
South Beach diet, 19, 26
sour pickle spears, 154
stock. *See* soup
strawberries, 59, 76, 121
supermarket
    impulse buys, 100–101, 105
    layout, 43–44, 58, 100
sustainable agriculture, 88–89
sweet tomato jam, 157–58

tallow, 21
Thirty-Month Plan, 87, 99, 123,
    143–50

tomato powder, 133, 156
tomatoes, 59, 102, 106, 114,
    118, 120, 121–22, 129,
    133, 144, 157–58

U.S. Department of Agriculture
    (USDA), 41, 46, 80

vanilla extract, 123
vitamins, 24–26, 44, 49, 64
    B, 25, 64
    C, 64
    E, 25
    synthetic, 25–26, 65

weight
    health and, 16, 17
    media focus on, 16
Weight Watchers, 23
whey, 35–36, 49–50
whole grains, 19, 25–26, 52
work fulfillment, 6–7, 34

About the Author

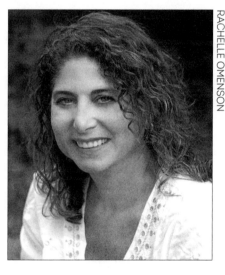

RACHELLE OMENSON

J. Natalie Winch lives in southern New Jersey, not far from where she grew up, with her husband, two children, and dogs. She currently works as a high school English teacher, for which she blames her own former high school English teacher Bobbi Katman, who was intelligent, inspiring, and cared enough to set very high expectations for her students. When she isn't mothering, teaching, grading, or making lesson plans, Natalie runs the Hebrew School at her synagogue, coaches soccer, teaches lacto-fermentation classes, writes the occasional entry for her blog Food Empowerment (trads notfads.com), and fights the dust bunnies that threaten to take over her family room.